Forensic Pathology Basics

The Dead Do Tell a Story

by Dr David Holding

First published by
Words are Life, 2021
www.wordsarelife.co.uk

First published in Great Britain in 2021 by
Words are Life
10 Chester Place,
Adlington, Chorley, PR6 9RP
wordsarelife@mail.com
www.wordsarelife.co.uk

Electronic version and paperback versions available for
purchase on Amazon.
Copyright (c) Dr David Holding and Words are Life.

First edition 2021.

*"Hic Mortui Delectunt
Viventes Educere"*

*"Here The Dead Delight
to Teach the Living"*

Acknowledgements

I am very grateful for the support and encouragement I have received from numerous sources in the preparation of this work. In particular, I wish to express my thanks to the medical staff at the Lancashire Teaching Hospitals NHS Foundation Trust, and Manchester University Medical School, for the benefit of their expert opinions on issues raised in this work, and for their helpful suggestions. My appreciation also extends to the ever-obliging staff of the libraries and institutions I have consulted during my period of research.

Finally, my ever-grateful thanks must go to my publisher, Lesley Atherton. It is Lesley's unfailing support of my work, especially during this uncertain time, that has been a beacon of hope, providing the impetus and encouragement to drive me forward. Her enthusiasm and love of words never fails to impress me.

Dr David Holding, 2021

About the Author

Dr David Holding studied history at Manchester University before entering the teaching profession in the 1970s. He taught in both state and independent sectors. It was during this time that he continued historical research culminating in the award of both a Master's degree and Doctorate.

Having previously studied law, David gained a Master of Laws degree in Medical Law, which enabled him to transfer to teaching legal courses at university. Since retiring, David has concentrated his research and writing on various aspects of local history, legal trials, forensic science and medico-legal topics.

Also By David Holding

Murder in the Heather: The Winter Hill Murder of 1838
This book is a unique account of a brutal murder which occurred on the summit of Winter Hill in Lancashire in 1838. The account draws on both contemporary media reports and court transcripts and examines the events leading up to the killing of a 21-year-old packman. It details the proceedings of the trial of the only suspect in the case. The work concludes with a re-assessment of the case in the light of modern forensic investigation. The reader is invited to reach their own 'verdict' based on the evidence provided.

The Pendle Witch Trials of 1612
The book provides readers with a sequential overview of the famous chain of events which ultimately led to the execution of women accused of practising witchcraft in the county of Lancashire. It is presented as a chronological account of the famous trials at Lancaster Castle in 1612. The reader is introduced to all the evidence and interview transcripts that formed the major plank of the prosecution case in this book that will appeal to both the general reader and local historian.

The Dark Figure: Crime in Victorian Bolton
This book provides an absorbing overview of crime in the Lancashire town of Bolton over the period 1850 to 1890. It is primarily based on documentary survey and analysis of court and police records covering

the period. It assesses changes in crime over time and asks whether these relate to economic, social or political changes taking place at the same time. The reader is left to reflect on whether crime in all its many forms, has actually changed over time.

Bleak Christmas: The Pretoria Colliery Disaster of 1910
This work charts the events of the Lancashire Pretoria Pit disaster in December 1910. It reflects on the devastation it left to many of the local communities whose main source of employment was coal. The main sources analysed are the Home Office Report into the disaster and the Report of the Inquest. The findings of these detailed legal reports are presented in a format that will supplement existing material on the event. The book will also provide a reference source for both local historians and the general interested reader.

Doctors in the Dock: The Trials of Doctors Harold Shipman, John Bodkin Adams and Buck Ruxton
This book takes the reader on a journey into the world of three medical doctors in England, each coming from a different social background but with one common thread going through their lives. They all stood trial for murder. In each of the cases, the reader is involved from the start and presented with all relevant evidence available to jurors in the case. The overall aim of this work is to invite readers to exercise their judgment in reaching a verdict.

Forensic Science Basics: Every Contact Leaves a Trace
Starting from the basic principle of forensic science, this work is an absorbing introductory study of the techniques familiar to us all from numerous trials, media reports and TV crime dramas. The book examines such aspects as the time of death, causes of death, weapons of crime and identification of offenders and much more. It provides essential reading for those who wish to gain a basic introduction to this fascinating area of science.

A Warning from History: The Influenza Pandemic of 1918
The 1918 Influenza Pandemic was one of the most deadly events in human history, and understanding the events and experience of 1918 is of great importance to pandemic preparation. This book aims to address questions concerning pandemic origin, features and causes, and to provide the reader with an appreciation of the 1918 pandemic and its implications for future pandemics. This work will cater to both the science-orientated and general reader in this crucial area of global and

public health.

The Lady Chatterley Trial Revisited

The 1960 obscenity trial of Lady Chatterley's Lover remains a symbol of freedom of expression. It is also a seminal case in British literary and social history and credited as the catalyst which encouraged frank discussion of sexual behaviour. This book introduces readers to the trial itself, describing the prosecution and defence opening and closing speeches to the jury, and much more, before culminating in the judge's summin-up of the case, and the final verdict. The reader is provided with all the evidence to reach a considered assessment of the case and a question to consider – Can certain literature 'actually' corrupt, or does it simply encourage expensive court trials and boost sales?

The Oscar Wilde Trials Revisited

It is only given to very few people to be the principal figure in three Old Bailey trials, before three different judges, and at three consecutive court sessions, all in one year. This is one of the fascinations of the Oscar Wilde trials of 1895. In addition, they embodied celebrity, sex, humorous dialogue, outstanding displays of advocacy, political intrigue, together with issues of art and morality. Wilde's prosecution of the Marquess of Queensberry from criminal libel, and later, his own prosecution for 'gross indecency', reveal a complex person at odds with a class-centred and morally ambiguous Victorian society. This work considers these famous trials in chronological sequence and invites the reader to participate as both observer and potential juror in the proceedings. Finally, the reader is encouraged to consider the evidence presented at each of the trials, to arrive at their own conclusions. This work will be of particular interest to law students in regard to the advocacy skills so skilfully demonstrated by the respective counsel. It also caters for the general reader with a particular interest in the presentation of criminal cases in the courts in England.

The Whitechapel Murders of 1888

The killing of five women in the Whitechapel area of East London in 1888, remains the greatest and most horrendous of all unsolved murder mysteries. It is the classic 'Cold Case'. This work takes a novel look into the case from the perspective of the criminal investigation itself. In this approach, the more speculative and conspiracy theories that have surrounded the 'Jack the Ripper' crimes have been avoided. The reader is offered insights into these murders by employing the modern forensic techniques of geographical and offender profiling which shed new light on these serial killings.

Contents

Dr David Holding

Introduction

Forensic pathology has been defined as "the application of medical and scientific knowledge to determine the 'cause' and 'manner' of death". An alternative definition has also been proposed: "a field of forensic science which involves the application of pathological methods in the investigation of crime, and of sudden, suspicious or unexplained deaths".

However it is defined, forensic pathology is in many ways like a jigsaw puzzle. The pathologist finds on or inside a dead body, something unusual, which he or she must consider in reconstructing events concerning the death of the deceased.

It was only towards the middle of the nineteenth-century that forensic pathology really came into its own as a 'sub-speciality' of medicine. The English doctor, Alfred Swaine Taylor, wrote extensively on forensic pathology and helped to modernise the discipline within medicine in Britain. His most important textbook; *A Manual of Medical Jurisprudence,* published in 1831 went through ten editions during his lifetime. By the mid-1850s, Taylor had been consulted on more than 500 forensic cases.

During the late twentieth-century, there was a huge public demand for insights into the work of forensic pathologists. Influenced by this demand, not surprisingly, television companies became keen to capitalise on this emerging public interest. As a result, they began producing medical dramas based on the activities of fictional forensic pathologists.

One of the first of these dramas was the American *Quincy ME*, first appearing in the US in 1976 and in the UK in 1977. It was not until the 1990s that the UK produced its own medical dramas. One example is the BBC's *Silent Witness* which spanned the years 1996-2008.

The popular and successful dramas were replicated

in fiction, the most notable being the books by Patricia Cornwell in the 1990s. The downside of these fictional representations has been to confuse 'pathology' with 'forensic pathology' in the public imagination. However, to off-set this uncertainty, today's forensic pathologists have begun to utilise the medium of television to present a more realistic approach to their important work.

One excellent example came from Dr Richard Shepherd, a prominent forensic pathologist in the UK. He presented a 2006 series for the BBC titled *Death Detective*. The series focussed on the more routine coroners' cases rather than on violent crime.

It was equally important that it also included interviews with families of the deceased. They discussed openly the impact of the death on them, and were provided with explanations of how the Dr Shepherd's pathology findings helped the relatives to come to terms with their loss. Dr Shepherd's series, whilst confirming the association of pathologists with death, also provided a more realistic perception of their important work. It also emphasised the contribution that histopathology plays in the treatment of the living.

This work introduces the reader to the role that forensic pathology plays in determining the cause of death, and in confirming the cause as being the result of homicide, suicide, accident or natural causes. Each of the five chapters in this work provides informational continuity.

Chapter One provides an overview of the UK's existing legal systems, within which forensic pathologists have to operate.

Chapter Two discusses the most controversial aspect of forensic pathology and medicine – calculating the 'time of death'. It describes the various techniques that are applied to establish the time of death.

Chapter Three introduces the reader to the autopsy or post-mortem examination itself, the sequence in which they are conducted, and the compilation of the final report for the Coroner, outlining the main findings of the examination.

Chapter Four is devoted to an examination of the manner and cause of death, and describes in some detail, the various forms of criminal wounding, accidental injury and suicide.

The final chapter concludes with a collection of case studies, each describing the various causes of death discussed elsewhere in the text. This will assist the reader to appreciate the practical application of pathological theory.

A glossary of medical terminology is provided to help clarify many of the terms that appear in medical and post-mortem reports. In addition, a selected bibliography is included to assist readers interested in pursuing further research into the various aspects of forensic pathology.

The main objective of this work has been to reflect the status that forensic pathology now commands in the field of criminal investigation. It provides a compelling insight into the work of the forensic pathologist, and is recommended to all interested in the realities of detection, of which forensic pathology is a major player.

Chapter One: First Principles

The origin of the word *forensic* stems from the Latin *forum* and refers to matters of law. In ancient Rome, the town 'forum' was the centre where public trials were held, and justice dispensed. The modern term 'forensic' refers to science that is applied to matters of the law and in particular, to the criminal justice system.

Any branch of science contains a 'forensic' element. For example, forensic 'entomology' is concerned with the interpretation of insect infestation at the scene of a crime. Similarly, forensic 'odontology' refers to dental aspects of a crime, particularly the presence of 'bite marks' on a body, and to the identification of a body through the interpretation of the teeth.

The word, *pathology* comes from the Greek *pathos* meaning 'suffering'.

Linking the two words into the phrase 'forensic pathology' indicated that branch of medicine concerned with the structure and functional changes in human body tissues brought about by either disease or injury.

Finally, *disease* is defined as 'any alteration from normal health caused by injury or infection that can result in death'. So, *forensic pathology* can be defined as 'the branch of medicine that is concerned with the legal aspects of injury to the body that can result in death'.

From a practical point of view, forensic pathology is concerned essentially with the pathology of intentional (homicidal or suicidal) and unintentional (accidental) trauma or injury in cases where bodily damage may be the major contributory factor, and in death from 'natural' causes when the cause of death cannot be determined.

The Role of the Forensic Pathologist

Forensic pathologists are independent practitioners who provide 'impartial' legal opinions to police, lawyers and courts. In England and Wales, forensic pathologists providing services to police forces are registered by the Home Office Pathology Delivery Board, who maintain a Register of Forensic Pathologists.

They perform medico-legal autopsies (post-mortems) on behalf of HM Coroners in England and Wales and Northern Ireland, and for the Procurators Fiscal in Scotland. They also provide a service to police authorities in cases of suspicious death, and assist in the collection of forensic evidence at scenes of death. While some forensic pathologists are self-employed, others are employed either full or part-time in the NHS or at a university.

Their services are usually arranged by contracts for the pathological investigation of suspicious deaths which fall within a specific geographical area of the country. These pathologists work within 'group practices' composed of at least three pathologists. These groups provide a forensic post-mortem service 24 hours a day, and utilise specific mortuary facilities, although some still perform investigations in hospital mortuaries.

A forensic pathologist is a medically qualified practitioner registered by the General Medical Council (GMC in the United Kingdom). Those wishing to specialise in forensic pathology undertake post-graduate training in 'histopathology' – the study of the effects of disease on the human body. Following this foundation programme, progress is determined by the successful completion of the Royal College of Pathologist (RC Path) examinations. The whole process to qualifying as a forensic pathologist can take around six years to complete.

The duty of the forensic pathologist is to provide

15

answers to four questions for the coroner:
1. Who is the deceased?
2. Where did they die?
3. When did they die?
4. How did they die?

Forensic pathologists attend crime scenes at the request of the police. Their specific role is to make a medical assessment and advise on the medical aspects of an investigation. They also attend court to give evidence in criminal cases.

The pathological 'process' involving injury or disease ultimately leading to a person's death, is referred to as the Mechanism of Death. This can be a bullet wound to the head, a stab wound to the body or ligature strangulation.

The Manner of death refers to the particular circumstances surrounding a particular case of death. This can include homicide, accident, natural, suicide or undetermined death. This constitutes the How? of forensic pathology, and the Cause and Manner of death can be distinguished. For example, the 'cause' of death can be something like 'heart failure', whereas the 'manner' of death may result from a stabbing to the heart. In this sense, the 'manner' of death is the 'cause' of death.

Another way of expressing this in relation specifically to violent death, is that the 'manner' of death or the way the victim died can be a natural death, a suicide or a homicide.

Homicide is a descriptive epithet which means the 'killing of one person by another'. From a purely legal point of view, it can be murder, but also manslaughter or even self-defence. In this respect, 'homicide' is a more general term. In contrast, *murder* is a specific legal term implying 'intent' on the part of the perpetrator.

Forensic pathologists are not detectives but they use their knowledge and experience to assist the police in solving a case which involves death or injury.

For a forensic pathologist, involvement begins with a request from the police to look at a dead body. At that stage, the police may not know who the dead person is, and will need to be informed of any details that can help in the identification of the deceased. They will also want to know the cause or manner of death. Was it due to natural causes or to violence? If the latter, is it a case of accident, suicide or murder? This is vitally important if it is murder, and a suspect claims an alibi for the crime.

The forensic pathologist may be called on to give evidence either for the prosecution or the defence in a criminal trial. A forensic pathologist's involvement in an investigation may include visiting the scene of a death. They will gather information concerning what happened at the time of death, together with the medical history of the deceased person.

The pathologist will be 'briefed' as to the circumstances surrounding the case by the police Senior Investigating Officer (SIO). An *in situ* examination of the body will take place, noting its disposition, the surroundings in which the body lies, and the presence of any obvious injuries – all without disturbing the body or the scene.

The important rule here is that the body must not be touched until all photographs have been taken. The body itself must be lying <u>exactly</u> as it was when discovered. Under no circumstances should it be moved, turned or searched before the forensic pathologist has inspected it. Premature handling alters the body's original position. More importantly, it can leave foreign fingerprints, disturb organs, and change the balance of the body's inner fluids. Such actions degrade the body's forensic credibility. Any photographs taken of such disturbed body, will be counted as unreliable.

More importantly, the body is the prime evidence at any crime scene. By altering it original conditions, a pathologist's photographs may be declared 'inadmissible' evidence at any subsequent criminal trial.

The pathologist will supervise recovery of the body by funeral directors and direct that the body is transported to the mortuary for the medico-legal autopsy.

Medico-Legal Systems of Death Investigation in the UK

In the United Kingdom there are three independent legal systems for dealing with the way in which deaths are investigated. These systems operate in England and Wales, Scotland and Northern Ireland independently.

England and Wales – The Coronal System

The English office of Coroner was first mentioned in an ordinance of 1194, which required every Shire in the kingdom to elect an officer to "...keep the Pleas of the Crown".

The Statute *'De Officia Coronatoris'* of 1276, stated the Coroner's duties and obligations. The title of Coroner is derived from the original Latin *Custos Placitorum Coronae*, translated as 'Keeper of the King's Pleas'.

The medieval Coroner's judicial role included inquiring into matters of unexplained deaths. The Statute of 1276, together with its subsequent repeals and amendments, was eventually replaced by the Coroner's Act of 1887, which restated and defined the duties of the office of Coroner.

Following the Coroner's (Amendment) Act of 1926, a person is only eligible for appointment to the office if they are either a solicitor or barrister or medical practitioner of at least five years experience. Today, most coroner posts are held by solicitors, the appointment being on a part-time basis. However, in the large towns and cities in England

and Wales, full-time Coroners are appointed. Many of these are qualified in both medicine and law.

The procedure under which deaths are brought to the attention of the Coroner is well-defined. Every death in England and Wales, must be certified by a Registered Medical Practitioner as to its cause. The certificate is then deposited with the local Registrar of Births, Marriages and Deaths. If there is any suspicion surrounding the nature of the death, the Registrar is legally obliged to inform the Coroner. He or she will then decide whether to hold an Inquest.

There is no statutory duty upon a medical practitioner to notify any death to the Coroner. The law is satisfied once the doctor issues a Death Certificate. It is solely the Registrar's duty to inform the Coroner if any doubts arise. However, if a doctor has any suspicions regarding a cause of death, it is common practice in England and Wales for them to advise the Coroner directly.

Such suspicious circumstances fall into twelve categories.

1. Where deaths are sudden or unexpected, and where the doctor cannot certify the actual cause of death; or where the doctor has not attended the deceased during their final illness, or within fourteen days prior to their death.
2. Abortions, other than natural abortions.
3. As the result of accidents or injuries which contributed to the cause of death.
4. Deaths occurring under anaesthetics and following surgical operations.
5. As a result of a crime or suspected crime.
6. As a result of the use of drugs.
7. As a result of starvation or neglect.
8. Industrial diseases arising from the deceased's employment.

19

9. Deaths if unusual or suspicious.
10. Deaths occurring in police custody or prison.
11. As a result of poisoning from any source.
12. Where the cause of death is unknown.

On receipt of a doctor's concerns regarding a death, the coroner has two options available to him/her.

They can decide that no further action is necessary. In this case, the registrar will be notified to accept a certificate of death from a medical practitioner.

The second option would be for the coroner to order an autopsy (post-mortem) examination. This would be in order to establish the cause of death if this is not obvious. A Post-Mortem Examination Report will be completed by the pathologist and given to the coroner. The coroner may then dispose with an inquest if he/she believes it to be unnecessary, and there is no reason to suspect that the person died a violent or unnatural death. The body of the deceased will then be released for the funeral, and the death registered by the registrar.

However, if the death was not due to a 'natural' cause, the coroner will hold an inquest. The inquest is a limited fact-finding inquiry to establish answers to the following questions: who died, when and where the death occurred and how the cause of death arose.

An inquest is usually opened to record that a death has occurred, to identify the deceased, and to issue documents required for burial or cremation. The inquest will then be adjourned until any police enquiries and Coroner's investigation are complete – at this point the full inquest can be resumed. The inquest is not a trial, but an inquiry into the facts surrounding a death. The coroner does have the power to investigate not just the main cause of death, but also "any acts or omissions which directly led to the cause of death".

Following an inquest, the coroner may arrive at one

of the following conclusions:
1. Killed Unlawfully.
2. Killed whilst the balance of his/her mind was disturbed.
3. Accidental/Misadventure.
4. Natural Causes.
5. Open verdict.

Once the conclusion has been reached by the inquest, the coroner provides the registrar with a certificate including the circumstantial, as well as the medical causes of death. Most inquests are held without a jury. However, in certain circumstances, the coroner must sit with a jury if it appears that there is a reason to suspect that one of the following criteria is satisfied:
1. The death occurred in prison.
2. The death was caused by an accident, poisoning or disease which requires notice being given to a government department, eg: deaths on railways, accidents on board British ships, or involving civil or military aircraft.
3. The death occurred in circumstances which is prejudicial to the health and safety of the public.

Scotland – The Legal System

Scots law was independent of England until the Act of Union in 1707. However, this Act still made provision for retaining a separate legal system to that of England. Criminal law in Scotland is administered by a Public Prosecutor, the prime holder of this office being the Lord Advocate. He, together with the Solicitor-General and Advocates Depute (collectively known as Crown Council), prosecute on behalf of the Crown, for the High Court of Judiciary. These officials preside in Edinburgh, but also sit on a regular Circuit of the major cities in Scotland.

The Procurator Fiscal

The Procurator Fiscal is appointed by the Lord Advocate and must be a practising lawyer. One is appointed for each of the Sheriff Court Districts in Scotland. The Fiscal is comparable to the office of Public Prosecutor in many continental legal systems.

This role includes the investigation of sudden, unexplained or suspicious deaths, and the main concern is in excluding any criminality. To achieve this, the proscurator fiscal requests either an external medical examination or a post-mortem to be performed by a forensic pathologist.

The essential function of the fiscal is to receive reports from the police on all crimes committed in his district, and to direct the police in their investigation. In addition, the fiscal also conducts prosecutions in the Sheriff Court, and prepares the crown case in a criminal trial committed to the High Court.

In death investigations, it is the primary concern of the fiscal to establish whether or not there has been any crime or possible negligence involved in a reported death. This function in death investigation is similar to that of the English coroner. However, the procurator is not obliged to establish the precise <u>cause of death,</u> in the medical sense, once the possibility of criminal proceedings have been ruled out.

By contrast, the coroner must establish the precise cause of death. In England and Wales, approximately 25% of all deaths are referred to the coroner, with virtually all of these requiring autopsy. In Scotland, about 13% of deaths are referred to the fiscal of which about 70% require autopsy. The overall autopsy rate in England and Wales is approximately 25%, in Scotland about 9%.

The fiscal investigation of sudden death differs from the coronal system in that there is no routine public inquest. However, one may be held under certain circumstances. In Scotland, any doctor can certify death if he/she feels competent to do so. In England and Wales, only the doctor who was in attendance during the last illness may do so. As in England and Wales, the only person with a statutory obligation to report a death to the fiscal is the Registrar of Births, Marriages and Deaths.

However, in practice, most cases are reported directly to the fiscal by doctors and the police. It is the duty of the appropriate procurator fiscal to enquire into all sudden, suspicious, accidental, unexpected and unexplained deaths. When informed of a death, the fiscal may order further enquiries via the police. However, the police are unlikely to become involved in the majority of hospital deaths.

It is the fiscal who decides on the need for an autopsy. If the fiscal is satisfied that death is due to natural causes, and that there is no evidence of criminality or negligence, they will invite the doctor to issue a death certificate. If however, the fiscal considers that an autopsy is necessary on any of the following four grounds, he must apply to the sheriff for authority to perform the autopsy, which is very rarely refused.

1. The fiscal's enquiries cannot be completed unless the cause of death is fully established.
2. That there are circumstances of suspicion.
3. That there are allegations of criminal conduct.
4. That the death is associated with anaesthesia in connection with a surgical operation.

It is Crown Council who make the final decision as to what proceedings, if any, will follow a death. Not every death reported to a fiscal requires to be reported by him. Sudden deaths that in the opinion of the fiscal are free from suspicion, may be cleared up by him. However, there are certain categories of death which require to be reported to the Crown Office:

1. Where there are any suspicious circumstances.
2. Where there is a possibility that criminal proceedings may be instituted.
3. Where the circumstances point to suicide.
4. Where death is due to a medical mishap.
5. Any death of a member of the Armed Forces or a police officer resulting from an accident while on duty.
6. Deaths resulting from fire or explosion.
7. Any death resulting from abuse of substances.
8. Any death in which the circumstances are such that in the opinion of the procurator fiscal, the death should be brought to the notice of the Crown Council.

Crown Office may order further enquiries to be made if they are not satisfied with the conclusions of the fiscal's investigation. The Lord Advocate may decide that no further action is necessary, or may initiate criminal proceedings.

The Judiciary in Scotland

Criminal law in Scotland is administered by a Public Prosecutor – the Lord Advocate. Together with the Solicitor-General and twelve Advocates Depute (Crown Council), they prosecute before the High Court of Judiciary on behalf of the Crown. The Crown Office in Scotland, is the equivalent of the English Lord Chancellor's Department, but it also has a function of prosecuting, similar to the English Crown Prosecution Service (CPS).

Scotland is divided into six regions called Sheriffdoms, each with a Sheriff Principal who is responsible for the conduct of the courts. The Public Prosecutor in both the Sheriff and District Courts is the

Procurator Fiscal – a legally qualified member of the civil service whose role is to assess the evidence in each case, and then to decide whether or not to proceed with a case to trial.

Northern Ireland

In Northern Ireland, there is a Coronal System, which differs from that in England and Wales in a number of respects. Northern Ireland Coroners must be practising solicitors. The Coroner for Belfast is a full-time appointment and those for the other six counties are part-time appointments.

Section 7 of the *Coroner's Act (Northern Ireland) 1959* states:

"Every medical practitioner, registrar of deaths or funeral director, and every occupier of a house, mobile dwelling, and every person in charge of an institution or premises in which a deceased person was residing, who has reason to believe that the deceased died, either directly or indirectly, as a result of violence or misadventure on the part of others, or from any cause other than natural illness or disease for which he has been seen and treated by a registered medical practitioner, within 28 days prior to his death, or in such circumstances as may require investigation (including death as the result of the administration of an anaesthetic) shall immediately notify the Coroner within whose district the body of such deceased person is, of the facts and circumstances relating to the death".

It can be clearly seen that this Section of the Act places a duty on a majority of people, including doctors, to report such deaths directly to the Coroner. Section 8 of the same Act, provides for the involvement of the local police in the investigation of the circumstances of such reported deaths. The Northern Ireland Government provides a full-time forensic pathology service to assist Coroners in their investigations.

Chapter Two: The Time of Death

"When did the death occur?" is one of the most frequently asked questions in Forensic Pathology. There is a common perception that estimating the time of death is a routine process. In fact, it is probably the most difficult of all questions that arise in medico-legal investigations.

At a most basic level, at death the human body begins to cool down simply because the heart stops beating and blood no longer circulates throughout the body. Under 'room' conditions, a body will lose heat at the rate of approximately 1.5° F per hour for the first six hours following death. There will then be a slight slowing of cooling over the following twelve hours at the rate of between 1-1.5° F per hour. After approximately twenty-four hours post-death, the body temperature will have reached that of the 'ambient' or surrounding air temperature. The body will then under 'normal' circumstances feel cold to the touch approximately twelve hours after death.

There are, however, exceptions to this normal progression of body cooling. For example, if the deceased died as a result of asphyxiation (strangulation), or cerebral haemorrhage (bleeding on the brain), the initial temperature at the time of death may well be raised above the normal temperature range of between 98.4 and 98.6° F.

It is well understood that a naked body will cool more rapidly that that of a clothed body, or one immersed in water. Also, a larger-built person will lose heat more slowly than a slight built person.

It is normal practice in forensic medicine to establish the body temperature of a dead body *in situ* before removal to a mortuary. Also the ambient temperature at the scene of the discovery of a body is taken to establish a relationship between the two. A recurring problem for the forensic pathologist is the requirement to establish the 'time of death' within the limits of *probability* and not certainty.

27

Consequently, the more time that has elapsed between death and the time of discovery and medical examination of the body, the more extensive are these limits of probability.

From a legal point of view, the time of death is significant in relation to the questions of *alibi and opportunity.* For example, if a suspect can prove that he or she was at some other location when the fatal injury was inflicted on the deceased in a murder investigation, then they have an alibi, and their innocence is implicit.

On the other hand, if at the time of a fatal assault, a suspect was known to have been in the vicinity of the victim, then the suspect had the opportunity to commit the offence.

Algor Mortis

Algor Mortis (the medical definition for body-cooling) is the most useful single indicator of the time of death during the first 24 hours after death. The assessment of time since death is made by using calculations that use the body core temperature at the time of discovery of the body. The temperature is ascertained by using a rectal thermometer.

It is assumed that the body temperature at death was normal, which in most circumstances would lie between 96.7 and 99.0 degrees F.

The two important unknowns in assuming time of death from body temperature are (a) the 'actual' body temperature at moment of death, and (b) the actual length of the post-mortem interval between death and the examination of the body (usually in situ). It is for this reason that any assessment of time of death from body temperature cannot be accurate during the first three or four hours after death when these two unknown factors are most relevant. Body temperature cannot be a useful guide to time of death once the body reaches that of the ambient or surrounding temperature. Nevertheless, during the intervening period, any formula which involves an average of temperature cooling per hour, may provide a reasonably reliable estimate of time of death.

The most common method for determining a person's time of death using body temperature, is that of Moritz's Formula. This states that the body cools at a rate of approximately 1.5 degrees F per hour for the first twelve hours post-death, and then1degree F per hour for the next twelve hours. Assuming that the body temperature was normal at 98.6 degrees F, this figure minus the rectal temperature, is divided by 1.5 degrees F to give an approximate numbers of hours since death. For example, if the deceased was examined at 6:00pm and their core rectal temperature was 92 degrees F, then using the formula, it can be established that the person had died at approximately 1:36 pm that same day. The calculations would be as follows:

Normal Temperature	Core Rectal Temperature
98.6° F	92.0° F

$$1.5° F$$

The hours since death would be 4.4 hours. The numerator (upper figures) indicate how many degrees F the body temperature has decreased. In the example, a decreased of 6.6 degrees F is divided by 1.5 degrees F (the rate of cooling per hour for the first twelve hours, giving a figure of 4.4 – this being the approximate number of hours that have elapsed since death. To change the four hours to minutes, this is multiplied by 60 minutes per hour, which gives a figure of 24 minutes. The hours since death are subtracted from the time when the body temperature was first taken at 6:00 pm. This gives an approximate time of death at 1:36 pm.

A forensic pathologist would give an approximate

29

time of death based on the Algor Mortis calculations, plus or minus an hour either way, placing the time of death between 12:30 and 2:30 pm.

The reader can now appreciate that 'cooling' rate is the 'classic' method for estimating time of death, at least in the early stages of death investigation. However, it is important to remember that this method can only be applied in a maximum of between 20 and 24 hours post-mortem. There are however, other methods to be considered, that can be applied in conjunction with that of 'body cooling'.

Rigor Mortis

Death is followed immediately by total muscular relaxation known as *Primary Muscular Flaccidity*. This is followed by general muscular stiffening known medically as *Rigor Mortis*. After a variable period of time, Rigor Mortis passes off spontaneously. This is then followed by *Secondary Muscular Flaccidity*. These three stages are normally completed within a period of 48 hours after death.

When rigor is fully developed, the joints of the body become fixed. If a body is moved before the onset of rigor, then the joints will become fixed if the body is moved into a new position. If a body is maintained by rigor in a position that is not obviously associated with support of the body, it can be concluded that the body had been moved after rigor mortis had developed. This being the case, it would merit further forensic investigation.

It is generally accepted that rigor mortis passes off in the same order in which it develops. It begins with a stiffening of the eyelids about three hours after death, followed by the muscles of the jaw. The process then spreads progressively down through the face and neck, the chest and upper extremities, the trunk and then finally the lower limbs. This process is generally completed in around twelve hours post-death.

In the majority of cases, the stiffening will have begun to wear off within about 36 hours after death. By 48 hours, the body will have returned to secondary muscular flaccidity. In temperate climates, rigor will typically start to disappear about 36-48 hours post-death. However, if the environmental temperature is high, then the development of putrefaction (decomposition) will displace rigor within nine to twelve hours post-death. Also, advanced putrefaction as a result of the deceased suffering from septicaemia, will also lead to a rapid displacement of rigor.

Cadaveric Spasm

This is a form of muscular stiffening which occurs at the moment of death. Its cause is unknown but it is usually associated with <u>violent</u> deaths. It is of medico-legal importance because it records the last act in the life of the deceased. It most commonly involves specific groups of muscles, such as those of the forearms and hands. Should an object be held in the hand, then cadaveric spasm should only be considered if the object is firmly gripped and considerable force is necessary to break the grip.

Cadaveric spasm is seen in a relatively small proportion of suicidal deaths from firearms, incised wounds and stab wounds, when the weapon is firmly grasped in the hand at the moment of death. In such circumstances, the grasping of the weapon creates the presumption of self-infliction of the resultant injuries. This state cannot be reproduced after death by placing the weapon in the deceased's hands to replicate a suicide.

In cases of presumed drowning, it can be seen when grass, weeds and other materials are clutched by the deceased. In such circumstances, it provides proof that the person was alive at the time they entered the water. In cases of murder, hair and clothing from the assailant may be found in the hand of the victim.

31

Rigor mortis as an indicator of time since death, allowances must be made for the significant variations in the rate of onset and duration which can be wide. In general, if the body has cooled to the ambient (environmental) temperature, and rigor is well-developed, then it can be estimated that death occurred more than one day previously. Putrefaction or decomposition occurs about three to four days post-mortem in a temperate climate. Slight rigor can be detected within a minimum of 30 minutes after death, but it can also be delayed by up to seven hours. The average time of first appearance is three hours. It reaches a maximum of complete development after an average of eight hours, although this can take place as early as two hours after death or as late as twenty hours.

One rule of thumb offered by the late eminent English forensic pathologist, Professor Francis Camps was;

"Corpses can usually be divided into those still warm, in which the 'rigor' is still present, indicating death within about three hours.
Those in which 'rigor' is still progressing, death probably having occurred between two and nine hours previously. Those in which 'rigor' is fully established, show that death occurred more than nine hours previously".

Livor Mortis (Hypostasis – Lividity)

Lividity is a dark purple discolouration of the skin on a dead body, resulting from the gravitational pooling of blood in the veins and capillaries. This lividity is able to develop post-mortem because the blood remains liquid rather than coagulating throughout the vascular system. Within 30 to 60 minutes of death the blood in most corpses becomes permanently fluid. This is due to the release of fibrinolysins. This fluidity and lack of coagulation of the blood is a commonplace observation at autopsy.

Hypostasis begins to form immediately after death, although this may not be visible for some time. Its earliest appearance is as dull red patches on the skin of the corpse around 20 to 30 minutes after death although this timing can vary. These patches of livor then increase in intensity to reach a maximum extent on average within twelve hours (though there is great variation). The importance of lividity lies in its distribution as an indicator of body position and contact with objects, and in its colour, as an indicator of cause of death.

The usual purple colour of lividity reflects the presence of deoxyhaemoglobin. For this reason, the blood of a corpse becomes purplish-blue. This has to be distinguished from death from cyanide poisoning which also shows the pink hue of oxyhaeomoglobin. Carbon-monoxide poisoning produces the cherry red of carboxyhaemoglobin, while poisoning from sodium chlorate nitrates displays a grey-to-brown colour of methaemoglobin.

After about twelve hours, lividity becomes 'fixed' and repositioning of a body will result in a dual pattern of lividity, because the primary distribution will develop in the newly dependant parts. The blanching (whitening) of livor by thumb pressure is a simple indicator that lividity is not fixed. Well-developed lividity fades very slowly and then only incompletely. Duality of the distribution of lividity is important to medico-legal investigations because it shows that the body has been moved after death. For example, did the deceased die where the body was discovered or at some other location?

Putrefaction (Decomposition)

Putrefaction is the post-mortem destruction of the soft tissues of the body by the action of bacteria. Typically, the first visible sign of putrefaction is a greenish discolouration of the skin on the anterior (front) abdominal wall of the body. There is considerable variation in the time of onset and the rate of progression of putrefaction. Consequently, the time taken to reach a given state of putrefaction cannot be judged with any accuracy.

Under average conditions in a temperate climate, the earliest changes occur between about 36 hours and three days post-death. Progression to gas formation and bloating of the body occurs after about one week. The temperature of the body after death is the most important factor determining the rate of putrefaction. If it is maintained above 26°C (80°F), then the putrefaction changes become obvious within 24 hours, and gas formation is evident in about two to three days. In a hot humid environment with heavy insect activity, a corpse can be skeletonised in as little as three days.

All soft tissues are generally lost before the skeleton begins to disarticulate from the head downwards. Skeletal remains are of forensic interest only if the time since death is less that a human life-span of about 75 years. This is because any perpetrator of a crime could still be alive. Dating skeletons requires the services of the forensic anthropologist who can provide an investigation with details of the person in life. Interestingly, it is usual for the the bones of persons who died after the 1940s to contain high levels of Strontium-90 – acquired in life from atmosphere contamination caused by nuclear explosions.

Gastric Contents

If the last known meal is still present in the stomach of a corpse, and the time of that meal is known, this can give some general indication of the interval between the meal and the time of death. In general, if all, or almost all of the last meal is present within the stomach, then there is a reasonable medical certainty that death occurred within three to four hours of eating. Similarly, if half of the meal is present, then it is reasonably certain that death occurred not less than one hour and not more than ten hours after eating the meal.

However, these times are broad generalisations and difficulties arise in individual cases. This is because the biology of gastric emptying is complex, and is influenced by a wide variety of factors including the size and type of meal, drugs, stress and natural diseases. There have been several cases of alleged miscarriages of justice in which medical experts have wrongly used the stomach contents at autopsy, to provide estimates of time of death to an accuracy of 30 minutes, whereas the degree of accuracy is at least within a range of at least three to four hours.

Entomology

Forensic Entomology is the study of insect activity within a legal context. The most frequent application of this branch of forensic science, is to determine the minimum time since death, or the Post Mortem Interval (PMI) in the investigation of a suspicious death. This investigation involves identifying the age of insects present on a human body. Insects will quickly colonise a corpse, particularly one discovered outside.

The most important flies whose larvae (maggots) feed on corpses, belong to the groups 'Calliphoridae' – also known as blow-flies. These blow-flies are the bright blue and green 'bottle-flies', and are commonly found around discarded refuse. These female flies lay their eggs on the moist body parts such as the eyes, mouth and open wounds. After the adult fly has laid its eggs, they hatch within a few hours, depending upon the species and the ambient temperature. This commences the first of three precise stages or instars of development. These larvae feed on the corpse. When large masses of maggots are present on a dead body, they can generate considerable heat, and give off a strong odour of ammonia, their main excretory product. The post-feeding larvae (called prepupae) then migrate from the corpse to find a protected location in which to pupate. In due time, an adult fly will emerge from the pupa, and the life-cycle begins again.

For each species, this life-cycle follows a known temperature-dependant time course. Consequently, maggots of a known stage of development, and species that are found on a corpse, give an indication for the time required from their development or growth, of the minimum period since death of the corpse.

The pattern of corpse colonisation by successive waves of insects provides a source of further information. Moving a body and burying it some days after death interrupts the normal succession of insects. From this fact, it can be deduced that an event occurred to disturb the normal chain of events. Also blow-flies of certain species tend to be found within their preferred <u>urban</u> or <u>rural</u> habitat. Finding urban blow-fly larvae on a corpse in a rural setting suggests death took place in a urban environment, followed by the dumping of the body in a rural setting. This then raises suspicion regarding the actual circumstances surrounding the death of the person.

The larvae feeding on a corpse may may contain any drugs present in the actual corpse. These are often easier to analyse than body tissue because the corpse contains large numbers of chemicals produced by decomposition.

Botany

Plants and parts of plants may provide evidence of time since death, if a plant is in contact with a body or buried with human remains. A botanist will attend the scene of a suspected crime to inspect the presence of such plant.

Perennial plants such as trees, often have seasonal or annual growth rings, which can provide a minimum age for human remains where the plant or tree has grown through them. Annual plants give an indication of time because they complete their life-cycles in known time periods and in specific seasons. Disturbances that can be related to a point in the life-cycle of the plant can be dated.

Chapter Three: The Medico-Legal Autopsy

The terms *post mortem* examination which means 'examination after death', and *autopsy* meaning 'self-examination', are often used interchangeably in forensic medicine. In effect, there is no difference in definition.

Basically, a post-mortem or autopsy is a medical examination of a body carried out by a pathologist instructed by the coroner. The objective of this examination is to establish the 'cause of death' of the deceased, particularly when the death is unexpected or regarded as suspicious.

A full post-mortem examination involves examining each of the main body systems, including the brain and the contents of the chest and abdomen. This examination normally includes the removal and retention of small tissue samples for further examination under the microscope. Slides will be kept in a hospital pathology laboratory, and will form an integral part of a person's medical history.

The overall aim of the post-mortem is to provide answers to six questions; What happened To Who, When, Why, Where and How. On the completion of the examination, the pathologist will send a Report detailing everything found in the examination and the 'cause of death' to the Coroner and the deceased's GP.

In the investigation of a 'suspicious' death, the first task for the forensic pathologist is to examine the location in which the body of the deceased was discovered. It is here that vital evidence is collected which may have a direct influence on the case. The main concern of the pathologist is the actual position of the body, together with any body tissues or distribution of blood at the scene. During this initial examination of the body *in situ*, photographic records of the scene and body are essential, together with sketched plans of the location in relation to the position of the dead body. All these initial tasks are performed while the body remains 'untouched'. The relevant temperatures of the body and the surrounding air are taken. Both these are important as indicators of the time of death of the deceased.

Once these initial tasks are completed, plastic bags are placed over the hands and the head of the body and tied tightly. The rest of the body is wrapped in a plastic sheet and placed in a body bag for transport to the mortuary.

On arrival at the mortuary, the body must be identified and this can be achieved in three ways; <u>visual</u> identification by relatives and friends, <u>circumstantial</u> – by the way of papers, cards and identification documents found on the body, and <u>medical</u>, by teeth databases, x-rays and DNA samples.

The body is then weighed and measured and a brief description noted of the physical external characteristics of the deceased. The plastic sheet in which the body was wrapped is examined. It has been known for bullets to drop out of a corpse in cases of shooting during the transportation of the body from the crime scene to the mortuary. Any such objects found on the sheet are bagged, sealed and labelled.

While the body is still fully clothed, samples of both plucked and combed head-hair are taken, together with cuttings from the fingernails. The plucked hair also includes the 'root' which can reveal both the deceased' DNA and also the presence of drugs in the body.

The clothing is examined closely for the signs of any foreign material such as paint, grass, oil and blood. For example, a tiny smear of paint on the clothing of a road accident victim can be matched with the vehicle responsible for the injuries that led to the death of a victim.

In the past, it has been a routine practice to take a sample of the aqueous humour from the eyes of the deceased. This was because the level of *potassium* found in the liquid of the eyes rises in a straight line following death. This did prove quite an accurate measure of time of death, though it has now become a less used procedure because of its limitations in cases where there has been serious head injuries involving the eyes of the victim.

The next stage in the <u>external</u> examination begins with the removal of clothing from the body. Thr clothing is examined minutely for evidence of any damage. In particular, holes, tears, marks and discolourations are of importance to the pathologist, especially if any wounds are discovered on the body. The naked body is then examined in very great detail, usually beginning at the head and working downwards. Every inch of the skin is carefully checked for any obvious injury, bruise, scare and injection marks.

This is followed by a search of the scalp for any hidden wounds – and hair samples are taken. The mouth is examined for any evidence of tooth damage, toxic substances or cuts to the mouths or gums. The eyes are checked for evidence of *petechiae,* tiny specks of blood which are a common sign of asphyxiation.

All wounds found on the body are carefully measured and notes made of their precise location. For example, a stab wound to the chest can be described as 'being fifty inches from the ankle, and four inches on the left side of the midline'. The accuracy of these measurements can be crucial for matching up with the deceased's clothing, and also when presenting evidence in court at a criminal trial.

It is at this stage in the examination that temperature readings are taken again. In particular, notes are made of the stage of *rigor mortis* in the body, body staining as the result of the process of putrefaction, and the extent of lividity. When these tasks are completed, the <u>internal</u> examination of the body is ready to commence.

In most cases, and in all standard forensic examinations in the UK, a Y-shaped incision is made that begins with cuts behind each ear which descend roughly at

40

a 40 degree angle along the neck, meeting at the top of the chest, about the position of the sternum (breastbone). This incision then descends vertically to the pelvis area. This Y-shape incision allows for a better view of the larynx and throat. It also eases the procedure of pulling back the skin over the face to reveal the skull.

The internal organs are generally removed in blocks. For example, the heart and lungs may be removed together, and they would then be weighed. Thin slices are taken and preserved for microscopic examination. This is followed by opening the abdomen, when the stomach, spleen, kidneys and intestines are removed. These are individually weighed and examined for any damage or wounds.

The final stage of the internal examination is the pelvic region or cavity. The bladder is removed, urine samples taken, and swabs are taken as required.

Throughout the autopsy, the pathologist records every stage of the examination into a recorder and sometimes a video recording is also carried out. Photographs are taken of any significant details revealed during the autopsy. Tissue samples are taken from wounds, and in the case of fatal shootings, the bullet or bullets must be recovered from the body. In such cases, X-rays are taken to help reveal these.

The pathologist examines any broken bones, particularly in the case of suspected strangulation in which the *hyoid* bone in the neck will be fractured.

During the autopsy, the pathologist may also discover signs that suggest poisoning. Here the sense of smell is very important when it comes to the detection of substances such as ammonia or phenol (carbolic acid) in the stomach, or the characteristic 'bitter almond' odour of cyanide. Especially in suspected suicides, various chemicals may have been taken.

In one unusual case, a young girl was found dead in

41

her bed. At autopsy, on opening her skull, her brain gave off the odour of the cleaning fluid *Carbon Tetrachloride*. It was later discovered that she was in the habit of 'sniffing' the fluid.

The condition of the liver may indicate 'cirrhosis or hepatitis' or suggest an overdose of paracetamol. Inflammation of the kidney (nephritis) can be due to poisonous salts such as mercury compounds, lead-poisoning or long-term use of *phenacetin*. In gunshot wounds, swabs from around the wound can reveal powder residue. This can give a clue as to the range at which the shot was fired.

After completion of the autopsy, it is very important to reconstruct the body by reversing the dissection process. Where applicable, organs are returned to the body, or packing inserted where such organs have been removed for further analysis. The body is then firmly stitched. The aim is to provide both relatives of the deceased and funeral directors with aesthetically acceptable remains for the burial or cremation.

All autopsy reports conclude with the pathologist's commentary on the autopsy and its findings. This section of the report is interpretative and subjective in that it represents the opinion of the individual pathologist.

It includes the *cause of death* which will appear on the death certificate. The commentary brings together all the relevant information obtained from the examination of the body, the scene of death and the history of the deceased. Information obtained second-hand (hearsay) may be included from police reports, medical records and forensic reports. The relevant issues are addressed – What happened, to Who, When. Where, Why and How.

The length of commentary will vary in length as the circumstances dictate.

This information is directed to the Police Senior Investigating Officer (SIO) investigating the death, and to any other legally interested parties who may obtain access to the autopsy report. This commentary brings together the pathological autopsy findings and places them within the context of the whole case.

Autopsy Case Studies

The following case studies describe four separate UK autopsies on victims of violent crimes. These concern firearms-wounding, stabbing and blunt force trauma.

The case studies provide the reader with an insight into the 'investigative' role of the forensic pathologist in determining the 'cause of death' in cases of unlawful killing.

[1] Cause of Death : Gunshot Wounding

About twelve hours following a shooting, the victim's post-mortem took place. The deceased was described as being a male, six feet two inches in height, well-built and weighing thirteen stone, two pounds.

The back of his head revealed an entry wound, nine mm in diameter, two inches above and one inch to the back of his right ear. The left eye orbit had been destroyed by the exit wound. There was a second entry wound on the outer side of the left forearm also nine mm in diameter, and seven inches below the shoulder, with an exit wound on the inside of the arm and severely comminuted fractures of the left humerus. The bullet had passed clean through the arm, smashing the bone in its passage. Another entry wound was visible on the left side of the chest, and an exit wound one and a half cms in diameter surrounded by bruising, was visible five inches below the right shoulder. The second and third wounds had been caused by the same bullet.

The firearm used in this attack was described as being a nine mm self-loading pistol with a thirteen-round magazine. Two separate shots had been fired into the victim.

The scalp was bruised in the right parietal area, with fractures of the skull radiating from the entry wound in the right parietal bone across the vault of the skull and into the frontal fossa. The bullet had passed diagonally across the base of the skull, causing haemorrhage over the surface of the brain and destruction of the left frontal lobe, before entering the left orbit, destroying the left eye.

The lungs showed penetrating wounds on both upper lobes, caused by the bullet that had entered the left side of the chest between the second and third ribs on the right side. The trajectory of the bullet was exactly horizontal, fired at a man standing up and with his left side towards his assailant, perhaps beginning to turn away from, or even to turn towards his killer.

The heart was normal but the pericardial sac contained blood and the pericardium showed penetrating wounds. Crucially, the front of the ascending aorta had been severely lacerated. This would have been instantly fatal in this case.

[2] Cause of Death : Wounding by Stabbing

The victim was a male six feet three inches tall and well-built. There were small abrasions on the right side of the forehead and the right cheek, and a deep laceration half an inch long on the right cheek, extending down to the bone. There were further abrasions on the nose, slight bruising of the right upper lip, and a small bruise on the right side of the chin. The trunk showed three lacerations of a 'jagged' nature about half an inch long. The first was on the left side of the chest and had entered the chest cavity. The second was lower and to the left side, and had penetrated deeply into the muscles of the abdomen. The last was at the same height as the second but to the front right of the abdomen. It had penetrated the abdominal cavity but missed the organs.

There were abrasions on the front of the right knee, the left ankle, and the back of the right hand. The heart was normal in size and shape, but the pericardial sac contained a blood clot and there was a puncture wound at the apex.

The myocardium showed a laceration at the apex of the heart with an exit wound on the posterior wall of the left ventricle that had penetrated the internal chamber of the left ventricle.

There was a blood clot on the left side of the chest caused by the wound that had entered the chest cavity between the fifth and sixth ribs, cutting the costal cartilage of the sixth rib, two inches from the midline of the body. The victim had suffered four stab wounds. The first three to his cheek, his side and his stomach, would not have caused his death. The fourth however, went straight through his heart, travelling upwards and inwards and penetrating the main chamber.

Death would have occurred within seconds. In the opinion of the pathologist, a knife with a six-inch blade and about half an inch wide at its widest point would account for the injuries found on the victim.

[3] Cause of Death : Shotgun Wounds

The pathologist arrived at the scene of a shooting and found the body of a man lying face upwards on the ground. He was fully clothed and there were obvious wounds to his chest and neck. Rigor Mortis had not set in, and the body temperature was 34° degrees C (93.2° F), and he had not been dead long.

The body was removed to the hospital mortuary for the autopsy. On the front of the neck, just above the sternal notch, was a ragged hole ½ inch in diameter. Just below this and to the left was a slit wound again ½ inch long. On the left side of the chest were two circular wounds that passed inwards and upwards to enter at the first and second ribs. The back showed three circular wounds, each about ½ inch in diameter on the right side of the chest, all within a tight three inch radius. Internally, tissues on the right side of the neck showed severe bruising, the lungs showed penetrating wounds in the right and left upper lobes and around the root of the lungs.

The pleural cavities contained blood clots and blood on each side. There was a fracture of the fourth rib on the right side, and bruising in the right fifth interspace where a metal shot was found. A gunshot would have gone through the right scapula. Subcutaneous haemorrhages were present on the wall of the left ventricle of the heart, which was otherwise healthy, and there was bruising on the outer lining of the aorta.

X-ray examinations identified a further shot between the third and sixth thoracic vertebrae, where damage to the spinal cord had occurred, and further shot was removed from the right upper arm. The victim had received two distinct groups of injuries. The first, to the front of the chest, had passed upwards on the left side towards the right shoulder, with injury to the lung tissues around the shoulder and the neck, and penetration into the right upper arm. The second group was to the right side of the back, damaging the right shoulder blade, the spinal cord and the right lung.

Either of these groups could have caused death, but the back injuries were more severe and potentially more lethal. The victim had died from massive haemorrhage caused by shotgun wounds, having been shot in the back and through the chest.

[4] Cause of Death : Murder

The body of a thirty-year old male was discovered on the forecourt of his block of flats. This was reported to police who attended the scene, together with a police surgeon who confirmed life extinct. After initial investigation, it was assumed that the deceased had committed suicide by jumping from his fourth-floor balcony. This theory was supported by the discovery by police of a suicide note written in the deceased's own hand.

On further search being made of the property, a

knife was found in his bloodstained bathroom. Further examination of the body revealed slash marks on the man's wrists and neck.

Police enquiries revealed that the man had been depressed and had therefore decided to kill himself. It was assumed that he had firstly cut his wrists and then his throat, before finally jumping off his balcony.

At the request of the local coroner, the body was removed to the mortuary for an autopsy examination. Police photographs of the scene and of the body were made available for the forensic pathologist to study.

On examining the body, the first thing the pathologist noted was that the injuries found on the man's body were inconsistent with a fall from his fourth-floor balcony. There was a scalp injury to the area behind the right ear with associated skull fracture and brain damage. This particular injury did not appear to be consistent with the deceased having fallen from a height into the area in which he was discovered.

At this point in the autopsy, the pathologist studied the police photographs. In particular, he noted that in the kitchen of the deceased's apartment, one utensil was missing. In the bedroom, there was a heavy metal frying-pan lying on the floor, which aroused the pathologist's suspicion. The pattern of the head injury indicated that the man had either struck or was struck by a flat surfaced instrument. This would be typical of the effect from a heavy blow from such an object as the frying-pan. This injury would have rendered the man unconscious.

The severity of the bruising to the brain indicated that the injury was received some minutes prior to his death. As regards the slashing of the wrists and cutting of the throat, the pathologist noted that there were numerous, deep and superficial cutting wounds on the forearms and neck. These wounds were superficially consistent with self-inflicted injuries.

However, although these deep wound injuries were inflicted while the man was still alive, many of the superficial gouges appeared to have been caused <u>after</u> death. The pathologist's reasoning behind this was that the sheer number of wounds were far in excess of those seen in most cases of suicidal cutting.

The pattern of injury on the arms and parts of the legs was consistent with a fall from a <u>moderate</u> height but not consistent with a fall from a fourth-floor balcony. This conclusion was reached because of the lack of skeletal injury and deep muscle bruising which would accompany such a fall.

The pathologist concluded that the maximum height that he could have fallen from would have been from <u>one storey only</u>. The relative lack of bruising associated with these injuries indicated that he was already dead when he fell into the area where he was discovered.

The pathologist's conclusions indicated that the deceased did not kill himself, and that the likely scenario was that he was struck on the back of the head, probably with the frying-pan, and that this rendered him unconscious. He was then carried to the bathroom where his neck and wrists were slashed, resulting in severe haemorrhage. These cutting injuries were inflicted to mimic suicidal injuries. He was then removed from the bathroom and wrapped in some covering and thrown from a lower level in the block of flats.

The pathologist also noted something else in the police photographs. There had been a trail of blood on the tiled floor leading from the bathroom to the balcony. There was not enough blood, because the deceased would have bled heavily from the wounds on his body and this would have inevitably left a distinct trial of heavy bloodstains which were absent on the photographs.

The victim had a large bruise about six inches across on the back of his scalp, though there was not any skull damage. This was simply not consistent with someone jumping from a fourth-floor balcony.

Also, the cuts did not look like self-inflicted injuries. The method of inflicting them was wrong. They fanned <u>outwards</u> when they should have gone horizontally.

There was blood in the bath and a bloodstained knife by the side of the bath itself. These were not in the position where somebody would elect to cut themselves.

As the result of this autopsy, the police instigated a murder investigation. It later transpired that the victim had become involved in a domestic dispute with several individuals, who had gone to his flat. They had hit him on the back of the head with the cast iron frying-pan, knocked him unconscious then placed him in the bath. They then cut his wrists while he was still alive thus creating a trail of blood. Finally, they wrapped him in a carpet and took him downstairs to dump his body, where it was subsequently discovered.

The remaining question in this particular case is what would force a man to write a false suicide note?

Chapter Four: The Manner and Cause of Death

Wounds

A 'wound' can be described as anything that causes damage to the body's tissues. From a medical aspect, wounds and injuries are regarded as a single pathological entity. For the purpose of this work, 'wounds' are defined as injuries arising from an assault. Such wounds can be classified as blunt force injuries (bruises, abrasions, lacerations and bites), sharp force injuries (incisions and stab wounds) and gunshot wounds.

In England, the legal position regarding wounding is governed by the *Offences Against the Person Act 1861*. Section 47: *Assault Occasioning Actual Bodily Harm.* This is defined as "an assault resulting in actual bodily harm to another person"

Section 20: *Inflicting bodily injury with or without a weapon.* This is defined as 'unlawfully and maliciously inflicting grievous bodily harm upon another person, either with or without a weapon or instrument'.

Section 18: *Wounding with intent to cause grievous bodily harm.* This is defined as 'unlawfully and maliciously by any means whatsoever, to wound or cause grievous bodily harm to any person, with intent to do so'.

Blunt Force Injuries

[1] Bruises

The word 'bruise' comes from the Old English word *bryson* meaning 'to crush'. A bruise is defined as a leakage of blood from ruptured small vessels (veins or arterioles) into surrounding tissues of the body. Haemorrhage or bleeding is the escape of blood from any part of the

51

vascular system. In this respect, bruising is a form of haemorraging into surrounding tissues, and can be seen in surface skin, muscle or any internal organs.

Most bruising is due to <u>blunt force trauma</u> which can be a moving object striking a stationary body, such as a blow from a fist or weapon. Bruises rapidly appear at the site of impact. Bleeding into the subcutaneous tissue is seen as discolouration in the surrounding skin.

Any <u>internal</u> bruising is not visible on the surface of the skin. Bleeding into tissues may continue for some time following impact due to circulatory pressure. As a result, deep bruising may take up to 24 hours to appear on the surface of the skin. Bony prominences such as the shin, cheek and orbits surrounding the eyes will bruise easily.

The extent of bruising can be influenced by four other factors:

1. Age – Very young children and the elderly bruise much easier.
2. Obesity and Sex – Obese persons bruise more easily due to a greater proportion of subcutaneous fat. Females generally bruise more easily because they too, have a greater proportion of fat than males.
3. Disease of Clotting – Spontaneous bruising due to leukaemia, haemophilia and platelet disorders. Also persons of anticoagulant therapy.
4. Skin Colour – Black skin may mask bruising, but this can be revealed by the use of UV lighting

Age and Colour Changes in Bruises

At the time that the bruise was created, its initial colour will be <u>dark red</u> which is the colour of capillary blood, which then soon changes to <u>purple</u>.

All the subsequent colour changes in the development of bruises vary in respect to their timing. These colour changes start at the periphery (outer limits) of the bruise before progressing towards the centre, especially in the bruised area is relatively large. In the case of smaller areas of bruising, they may change colour more uniformly.

Colour Changes of Bruises
Dark red
Purple
Brown
Green
Yellow
Straw
Disappears (usually within fourteen to fifteen days but can range between one and four weeks).

Generally, a small bruise in a healthy adult may disappear in around one week. The time course is very variable, dependant upon the size and depth of the bruise, the site on the body, and on the age and general health of the individual. Accurate dating of an individual bruise is difficult, but distinguishing fresh from old bruises is easier. This is important forensically in cases of suspected repeat assaults and child abuse.

Patterns of Bruising

(a) Patterned Intradermal Bruise
This is usually due to impact with a hard patterned object with ridges and grooves. The resultant bruise may display the pattern of the object – for example, a vehicle tyre mark, shoe tread, car bumper or gun muzzle.

(b) Tram-line Bruising
These bruises are due to a rod-shaped weapon or stick. Traction causes rupture of the vessels along the edges of a rod. A flexible strap or belt will wrap around the body surface producing a longer and often curled tram-line

bruise.

(c) Doughnut Bruise

This is due to a <u>spherical</u> object such as a cricket or golf ball.

(d) Finger Pad Bruise

These are oval or round and are due to gripping by fingertips in forceful restraint. They are usually found on the limbs and face (in child abuse), the thighs (in rape) and the neck (in manual strangulation).

In examining bruises, it is it is useful for the pathologist to trace their outline onto an acetate sheet for later comparison with data charts. From a forensic view, the colour of bruises does not change after death, and they may become more evident against the pale skin of a corpse.

However, it is not possible to distinguish a bruise sustained at the time of death from one which occurred a few hours earlier. Such bruises are better described as having occurred 'at or about the time of death'. If a microscope examination of a bruise shows an inflammatory reaction, then it was likely inflicted more than a few hours <u>before</u> death.

Bruises to the deep tissues can be present without any evident skin surface injury. This is particularly the case if the force applied to the skin is by a smooth object over a wide area. Such deep bruises may spread under the influence of gravity and body movement. They follow the path of least resistance within the tissues. This shifting of deep bruises explains their delayed appearance at the skin surface some days after infliction, and often at sites distant from the original point of impact. For example, the delayed appearance of bruising around the eyes results from a blow to the forehead.

A second examination of a victim of an assault after

an interval of a few days, may well reveal visible bruising where previously there had been only the swelling of a deep bruising.

Deep bruising which amounts to haemorrhage may have severe, immediate or long-term effects. These are influenced by the function of the structure involved. A bruise within the eyeball may cause permanent blindness. Likewise, bleeding on the brain may cause irrecoverable damage to the nerve cells. Generally, bruises occurring in the subcutaneous tissue seldom cause serious damage unless they become infected.

[2] Abrasions

The word 'abrasion' derives from two Latin words; *ab* meaning 'from', and *radere* meaning 'to scrape'.The medical definition for an abrasion is "a portion of the bodies surface from which the skin has been removed by the action of 'rubbing'".

An abrasion occurs when the outer skin is damaged but the deeper layers remain intact. Although little harm is caused to the body by such abrasions, rupture of vessels of even minute size may result in the reproduction of the object that caused the abrasion.

Moving abrasions will not replicate the pattern of the object causing them, but will provide evidence of the direction of the abrasive force.

Parallel linear abrasions are suggestive of having been caused by fingernails. They may also confirm the fact of an assault having taken place, and provide evidence of the relative positions of the attacker and victim.

Impact abrasions without significant movement on the part of the victim, often reproduce closely, the object which caused the injury. Examples of these include imprints of weapons, and boots used in an assault. An outline of a contact object will appear where the skin having loose underlying connective tissue is struck. This causes the abrasion by the movement of the skin at the edges of the object.

Where the skin surface comes into contact with a rough surface, this results in grazing or scratch. This is the result of tangential friction.

Direct impact is where the skin is crushed, and is most often seen in fatalities.

[3] Lacerations

The term 'laceration' comes from the Latin *lacerare* meaning 'to tear'.The medical definition is a 'full thickness tearing of the skin due to the stretching, pinning or crushing of tissues by blunt force trauma'.

Lacerations can appear as three types; firstly, with ragged edges where the skin is torn apart, secondly, in combinations with bruising and abrasion, and thirdly, in tissue bridges in which there is a deep wound.

For example, a stellate laceration is one which radiates from a contact area, following a blow from an object such as the end of a poker. A linear weapon such as a stick will cause a linear laceration giving it a 'Y' shape. A hammer or other weapon with a circular striking face, will produce a circular or crescent laceration. Lacerations to the inside of the lips will result from the crushing of the lips against the teeth, following a blow to the mouth. Lacerations can be produced when the skin is stretched and the forces exceed the elastic limit of the skin. These tears or stretch lacerations are often seen on the groin of pedestrians struck from behind by a vehicle.

Extreme 'tangential' shearing forces, such as those produced by vehicle tyres when a pedestrian is run over, produce 'flaying' injuries with the raising of large areas of skin from their underlying soft tissues. The depth of a laceration often contains foreign material which is a source of wound infection. Blood and tissue recovered from a suspect object can be linked to the victim through both DNA profiling and blood typing.

[4] Bite Marks

Tooth marks inflicted on a victim can comprise abrasions, bruises or lacerations, or in some circumstances, a combination of all three. <u>Animal</u> bites tend to be deeply arched or 'u-shaped' whereas a human bite is more 'circular or oval'. It is the size of the mark which indicates whether it was inflicted by an adult or a child.

The shape of bite marks is affected by the release of the teeth from the tissue. Human bites may be revealed as a series of separate bruises or as a curved line of bruising. When these marks are fresh, they may provide useful forensic evidence of the assailant's identity.

The forensic pathologist will usually enlist the assistance of a forensic odontologist for expert opinion in cases of injury through biting. The size and shape of the dental impressions are influenced by such distinguishing features as missing teeth or displaced ones. Most countries including the UK, maintain dental databases of registered dental patients and their records which can be checked against those of a suspect.

Sharp Force Injuries

[1] Incised Wounds

The term 'incised' comes from the Latin *incidere* meaning 'to cut into'. The medical definition is 'a clean division of the full thickness of skin or tissue under the pressure of a sharp-edged instrument'. A incised wound is also one which is <u>longer</u> than it is <u>deeper</u>.

Sharp-edged instruments used to make an incision

can include a knife which is linear and clean, jagged metal which is irregular, or broken glass. The characteristics of an 'incised' wound are:

1. A clean cut with everted edges.
2. No tissue abrasions at the margins.
3. Linear or elliptical in shape which often gape open. Often deeper at the starting end.
4. Are more 'jagged' if inflicted on loose or folded skin.

Incised wounds are of forensic importance because they reflect the sharp edge of an instrument or weapon. There is profuse external haemorrhage with these wounds. The danger to life depends upon the site and depth of the wound. These wounds can also be self-inflicted, the result of an assault or accidental.

Most incised wounds are inflicted by the use of knives. The key feature of incised wounds reflects the fact that they are produced by sharp-edged objects. With incised wounds there is always <u>complete severance</u> of all tissues within the depth of the wound. Occasionally, incised wounds have irregular or ragged margins because the object used has an irregular edge (such as broken glass) or if the cut was made across skin folds such as the neck or palm of the hands.

Incised wounds inflicted with heavy-bladed instruments such as an axe, machete, meat-cleaver, hatchet or sabre all show abrasion and bruising of the wound margin. Also, the large size of the wounds and associated cuts are pointers that the weapon used in particular attack was <u>heavy-bladed</u>.

The ready availability of knives, together with the relative painlessness of incised wounds, have encouraged their use in suicide for a long time. Self-inflicted incised wounds are directed towards those parts of the body where large blood vessels are close to the skin surface, such as the neck and wrists. Suicidal incised wounds are very commonly accompanied by parallel, shallow, <u>tentative wounds</u>. These reflect a testing of the weapon, as well as indicating some hesitation on the part of the person. When healed, these wounds leave multiple, fine horizontal white scars.

Victims defending themselves against attacks with knives commonly sustain <u>defence wounds</u> to the hands and forearms. Defence wounds to the legs suggest that the victim was attacked while on the ground. In particular, cuts to the palms and fingers result from the victim attempting to grasp or deflect the weapon.

Slash or stab wounds to the back of the hands and forearms result from a victim's 'shielding' movements. The absence of defensive injuries would suggest that the victim was unable to offer a defence. This could be the result of the effects of alcohol and drugs, or if they had been rendered unconscious as a result of the attack.

Defensive wounds reflect <u>anticipation of injury</u> on the part of the victim, and their attempt to ward off the threatening harm.

Cleanly severed blood vessels within an incised wound bleed profusely, and if large vessels are cut, such haemorrhaging can be sufficient to kill. Such extensive haemorrhaging commonly results in blood soaking of clothing, together with staining and spattering of the location.

This does offer the possibility of reconstruction of the events through forensic <u>blood spatter analysis</u>. When large veins are severed, particularly in the neck, air may be drained into the circulation obstructing the flow of blood to the heart. Death would then be the result of <u>air embolism</u>.

[2] Stab Wounds

Stab wounds, like incised wounds, are associated with blood and tissue staining on the weapon, together with clothing. They also offer the opportunity for reconstruction of the events from an interpretation of blood spatter at the scene of the incident.

Stab wounds are essentially <u>penetrating</u> injuries which are produced by a long, thin object which is typically <u>pointed</u>. Most commonly, the object is flat with a sharp point such as a knife, a shard of glass, or a length of metal or wood. With sufficient force, even long rigid objects which are blunt-ended (such as a screwdriver) will produce <u>puncture wounds</u>.

The appearance and dimensions of the resulting wound often provide useful information regarding the object which produced the wound. The skin surface appearance of a stab wound is influenced both by the nature of the weapon and characteristics of the skin. The skin contains a large amount of <u>elastic tissue</u> which will stretch and recoil. This elastic tissue is not randomly distributed but aligned so as to produce natural lines of tension. These are known as *Langer's Lines.*

In survivors of knife assaults, the extent of the wound scarring will be influenced by the alignment of the wound relative to Langer's Lines. Wounds which have a long axis parallel with Langer's Lines, gape only slightly. Surgeons make use of this factor by aligning their incisions to promote healing and reduce scarring. However, wounds aligned at right angles to Langer's Lines tend to gape widely and scar prominently, because the natural lines of tension of the skin pull the wound open.

One important purpose in examining stab wounds is to establish whether potential weapons could have or could not have produced the wounds. The dimension of a stab wound give some indication of the dimension of the blade of the weapon. For example, if a stabbing with a knife is straight in and out, then the <u>length</u> of the stab wound on the skin surface will reflect the <u>width</u> of the knife blade. However, there are important qualifications that apply here.

The skin wound length may be marginally shorter than the blade depth because of the elastic recoil of the skin. For example, if the knife blade has a marked taper, and the entire length of the blade did not enter the body, then the skin wound length may not represent the maximum width of the blade. Also, if the blade did not pass straight in and out, but instead there was some rocking of the blade, or if it was withdrawn at a different angle to that of the original thrust, then the skin wound will be <u>longer</u> than the inserted blade width.

As a result, the most reliable assessment of blade width is made from the <u>deepest</u> wound with the shortest skin surface length. This is because this wound represents the greatest blade penetration with least lateral movement. A single weapon can produce a series of wounds which encompass a wide range of skin surface lengths and wound depths. This is most often seen in a <u>multiple stabbing</u> fatality, and is consistent with the use of a single weapon.

However, it is rarely possible to exclude the possibility of more than one weapon and, therefore, the presence of more than one assailant. As well as providing an indication of blade width and length, a stab wound may provide other useful information about the weapon. Wound breadth on the skin surface is a reflection of <u>blade thickness</u>. For example, a typical small kitchen knife with a blade thickness between one and two mm, will produce a <u>very narrow wound</u>. The use of a thicker-bladed weapon may be apparent from the measured wound breadth on the skin surface.

Most knives have a single edged blade, with one <u>keen</u> edge and one <u>blunt</u> edge to the blade. The thicker the blade of the weapon, the more obvious the blunting of one end of the wound when contrasted with that of the pointed end.

Knives with double-edged blades (daggers), are specifically designed for use as weapons. They produce a wound that is pointed at both ends. A hunting-type knife, having a rectangular metal plate between the blade and the handle, leaves rectangular abrasions. Weapons other than knives may produce different stab wounds. <u>Bayonets</u>, which have a ridge along the back of the blade, and a groove along either side to lighten the blade, produce wounds which are almost 'T' shaped. A 'forked' instrument (such as a garden fork) will produce <u>paired</u> stab wounds at different distances. A pair of scissors leaves paired wounds, pointed towards each other.

Stab wounds inflicted during a struggle, when knife thrusts are made at awkward angles, will reflect these movements between victim and assailant in the wound description. It is common for court proceedings to question the amount of force required to produce a specific stab wound.

It is usually difficult (if not impossible) to answer this question. It is the <u>sharpness</u> of the point of the weapon which is the most important factor in determining the degree of force necessary to produce a particular stab wound. In general, relatively little force is required to produce a deeply penetrating stab wound using a sharp pointed weapon. The greatest resistance to penetration is provided by the skin, and once this resistance is overcome, then the blade will enter the tissues quite easily.

To this end, the <u>depth</u> of the wound is not a measure of the degree of force applied during the stabbing. However, penetration of any bone does imply a significant degree of force having been applied. This is certainly the case if the tip of the blade has broken off and remains embedded in the bone. This will only become apparent when x-rays are undertaken.

The Mode and Cause of Death from Wounding

Rapid death resulting from incised or stab wounds is usually due to either haemorrhage or to damage to a structure that is essential to support life. Death may also be attributed to air entering a broken vein (embolism). Haemorrhage is by far the most common of these causes and will be much more severe if an artery is penetrated than if any veins are damaged.

The speed of death will largely depend upon the size of the vessel involved, and on the secondary effects of the accumulation of blood. It is difficult to inflict a stabbing injury of say fifteen cm (six inches) depth without laceration of an artery of at least moderate calibre. The direction of most homicidal stab wounds results in their frequent termination in the heart, aorta or major pulmonary vessels. Death in these circumstances is often very rapid.

Haemorrhage from non-penetrating incised wounds need not be severe unless a major artery lies superficially at the site of injury. The most obvious example is on the flexor surface of the wrist, which is a favourite site for suicidal incision. Rapid death due to interference with the function of structures other than blood vessels is rare.

For example, stab wounds at the nape of the neck, may result in near instantaneous death with minimal bleeding. This is due to the destruction of the vital centres of the medulla of the brain stem.

Incised wounds of the neck may result in many modes of death. These can be vagal inhibition of the heart, airways obstruction, air embolism, and bleeding from the carotid arteries.

Deaths attributable to wounds or injuries that occurred after the event, are usually the result of complications, such as pneumonia, pulmonary embolism or acute renal failure.

63

Survival Times after Wounding

Post-injury survival time is important in reconstructing criminal events. How long did the victim survive? And was the victim still capable of fighting, resisting or fleeing? These questions are commonly asked.

Some injuries are incompatible with any significant chance of survival. Any multiplicity of wounds which involve the heart and brain are associated with a short post-injury survival period. The effects of injury to major nerves, muscles and joints, followed by bleeding and shock, will ultimately incapacitate the victim. The time taken to do so, and what actions are still possible is very difficult to estimate. It has been suggested that, taken overall, 71% of stab-wound victims and 49% of gunshot victims survive for at least five minutes. However, when physical factors such as blood loss lead to immobility and loss of consciousness, death follows rapidly.

Gunshot Wounds

Shotguns can be either single or double-barrelled. They have a smooth <u>bore</u> or barrel, and are designed to fire multiple lead pellets or <u>shot</u>. The <u>calibre</u> or internal diameter of the bore of a shotgun is known as a <u>gauge</u>. This relates to the number of lead balls or pellets of a given bore diameter, required to make up one pound in weight. The most popular gauge is twelve, which represents a bore diameter of 0.729 inches (18.2mm).

The barrel of shot guns may be tapered towards the muzzle or barrel end, and fitted with a partial constriction known as a <u>choke</u>. The purpose of this is to restrict the spread of the shot once they are fired. Lead shot comes in a variety of sizes falling into two categories; <u>bird shot</u> which is used for birds and small game, and <u>buck shot</u> used for larger game.

The standard pellet sizes are designated by a numbering system. Individual cartridges bear the appropriate number to indicate the size of the shot contained within the plastic or cardboard cartridge. 'Bird shot' pellets range in size from 0.05 ins to 0.18 inches in diameter, while 'buck shot' range from 0.24 inches to 0.36 inches.

A shotgun cartridge consists of a plastic cylinder which is attached to a brass plate containing the 'primer' or powder source. This main powder charge is separated from the shot by a 'wad' or washer. When fired, the pellets are propelled out of the cylinder in a solid mass which then begins to fan out once it leaves the barrel. The propellant continues burning as the shot passes down the barrel, and some powder always remains unburned. The effective range of a sporting shotgun is approximately 50 yards, the shot being rapidly absorbed within the target structure.

Rifles and handguns have 'rifled' barrels which consist of spiral grooves cut into the length of the barrel. When a rifled weapon is discharged, this 'rifling' causes the bullet to spin. This increases its stability – and therefore the accuracy of the weapon. Handguns and rifles are the two most frequently encountered rifled weapons.

Handguns are designed, as the name suggests, to be fired from the hand, and consist of two types: revolvers and auto-loading pistols often referred to as 'automatics'. Revolvers have a revolving cylinder containing several bullets. On firing, the cylinder revolves around to enable all the bullets to be fired in sequence. 'Automatics' have a removable magazine holding a set number of bullets, which ensures auto-loading after each bullet is fired.

Rifles are designed to be fired from the shoulder, and consist of low and high-velocity models. A high-velocity bullet can travel at speeds of between 1,200 and 3,000 feet per second. At its maximum, this means that a bullet crosses the length of ten football pitches in a single second. Examples of such weapons include automatic pistols and service rifles. Bullets shot from low-velocity firearms such as a revolver, travel from muzzle to target at around 600 feet per second.

The Nature of Firearm Wounding

[1] Shotgun Wounds

A <u>contact</u> injury will show bruising due to the recoil of the gun, and a perfect representation of the single or double barrels may be found on the skin surrounding the wound. The shot will enter the body as a <u>solid mass</u> so that the <u>entry wound</u> will approximate to the <u>bore</u> of the barrel. However, explosive gases will also enter the wound so that the <u>external</u> wound may appear ragged and irregular.

If the target is the skull of a victim, it may be literally blown apart by the shot. If the site of the wound is the thick torso of the body, then an exit wound is unlikely, the shot having been absorbed and dispersed within the body tissue. Shot in its diffuse form as fired from a distance, has little penetrating power. Consequently, <u>exit</u> wounds are not a feature of shotgun injuries, other than in the context of a 'contact' shooting.

At very short range, the appearances will be modified by the effects of the gasses of combustion. Unburned powder will be discharged with the shot into the surrounding skin, leading to what is called tattooing, and soot is likely to be deposited around the wound. Hot gases will also scorch the skin and any clothing. These characteristics diminish as the distance from muzzle to wound increases. The critical distance is at about two yards (or metres), when tattooing is just about visible. After this distance, the shot begins to fan out creating a pattern of entry in the clothing and on the skin. The shot pattern will be circular, the size of this circle depending upon the degree of 'choke' of the gun.

There is a simple rule that can be applied to estimate the approximate distance between muzzle and target. The diameter of the shot pattern in centimetres is some two and a half to three times the muzzle distance from the wound. Alternatively, the spread of the shot pattern in inches is equal to the distance in yards. For example, if the shot pattern on a victim has a diameter of six inches, then the distance from which the shot was fired would be approximately six yards. Fatal twelve-bore shotgun injuries are unlikely at a range over twenty yards.

Effects of a Shotgun Wound Relative to Distance

Contact	Few inches	One yard
Ragged torn wound	Approximate one inch hole	Single entry hole
Burning and soot	Burning and soot	Tattooing
Tattooing	Tattooing	
Bruises		

Two yards	Six yards	Twelve yards
Irregular wound	Groups of pellets forming a 6-7 inch diameter	A uniform spread of pellets forming a 12-inch diameter
Pellet holes		

The majority of shotgun injuries are sustained at close range. Internal injuries are due to either the violent expansion of gas within the body, or to the penetrating effect of a <u>solid mass</u> of lead more than half an inch in diameter, entering the body. The former effect will be seen if the head is the target. The latter in the heart which can be torn apart by a shot fired within a range of two yards. With the exception of these two examples, the effects of a shotgun injury are variable and depend upon the ability of the individual pellets to penetrate internal organs.

[2] Rifled Weapon Wounds

The main difference between wounds due to shotguns and those from rifled weapons, is the fact that while shot will be found in the body of a victim, a bullet is very likely to have exited. Consequently, it is the <u>entry</u> and <u>exit</u> wounds that characterise wounds caused by rifled weapons. However, contact and close-range entry wounds display the same characteristics as those of a shotgun injury – bruising, blast effects, soot deposits and tattooing.

In the early phase of its flight, up to some 50 yards for a pistol and 150 yards for a rifle, there occurs considerable 'tail wagging' of the bullet which results in a relatively large and ragged entry wound. In the most efficient phase of flight, the bullet will enter the body nose on. This will leave a regular, small hole which, because of the elasticity of the skin, may very well not correspond exactly to the diameter of the actual bullet.

The entry wound will always show 'inverted' edges and likely to have 'soiling or contamination' by the grease covering the bullet which become wiped off by the clothing and the skin. As the bullet traverses the body, it may become deflected and deformed taking with it fragments of tissue, especially bone. These act as <u>secondary missiles</u> within the body itself. As a result, the exit wound is likely to be irregular and its edges everted.

The modern high-velocity rifle is something of an exception. This weapon kills as a result of the massive internal damage that results from the dissipation of large amount of 'kinetic energy'. The entry and exit wounds are relatively small and of similar size. The recovery of a bullet from the body is of vital forensic importance. Every weapon leaves a characteristic pattern of markings on the surface of the bullet.

Bullets may kill by virtue of penetrating the heart, a major vessel or a vital centre of the brain. By far the greatest damage is caused by <u>cavitation</u> in the track of the bullet, and by the discharge of energy which can tear vital tissues not necessarily in the direct path of the bullet. Delayed death is likely if a solid organ such as the liver is damaged. Also, death from septic shock or simple *sepsis*, may follow penetrating injuries to the stomach or bowel.

The Nature of Gunshot Wounds

In any case of fatal firearm wounding, there is always an immediate need to distinguish between accident, suicide or homicide. The medical evidence will depend ultimately upon an examination at the scene, and the findings of the post-mortem examination.

Initially, it is the scene of death which provides vital evidence in relation to suspected suicides. The weapon used must be within reach of the victim, and will either be retained in the grip or close to the hand of the deceased. A killer may attempt to simulate suicide, so it is important that the forensic pathologist notes the precise conditions of the body *in situ*.

The presence of the rare <u>cadaveric spasm</u> is of particular importance here. This is one post-mortem condition that cannot be artificially produced. Homicide is clearly indicated if the gun is found at the scene and is clearly beyond the reach of the deceased. Though, it is known that suicide can be achieved by means of a remote firing mechanism, such as a wire attached to the gun trigger.

Special note is made of the presence of spent cartridges in the case of shotgun wounding. The firing of more than one shot is very rare in cases of suicide. The

69

post-mortem findings indicating suicide are of vital importance. Findings indicative of a range within a yard, and the appearance of tattooing on the body, are clearly consistent with suicide. This is the maximum distance it is possible to hold a pistol from the body. The absence of close-range characteristics in a shotgun or rifle wound, will strongly mitigate against suicide because the barrel length of the gun approximates to that of the arm.

In practice, it is extremely uncommon for suicidal wounds to be other than of a 'contact' nature. They will also always be in a site of election. For example, a suicidal pistol wound is generally inflicted in the right temple, irrespective of the person being right-handed or not. An exit wound is usually close to the opposite temple. An alternative target is the centre of the forehead and the roof of the mouth. In either case, massive tissue damage can result. A rifle suicide may lean on the gun with the muzzle on the brow, or over the heart, a situation also seen in shotgun suicides. Two important features of successful suicidal firearms wounds are that they are always so placed as to eliminate the possibility of failure, and that the entry point must be accessible.

Certain features are strongly indicative of homicide; a single wound of contact or very close range type in an inaccessible position is obvious, the nape of the neck or behind the ear are obvious examples. Also the existence of more than one fatal injury will be very strong evidence eliminating either suicide or accident.

Case Study: Post-Mortem Report on PC Yvonne Fletcher, shot London, April 1984

Report by Dr Iain West – Home Office Forensic Pathologist

"X-rays taken before the post-mortem showed the absence of bullets or bullet fragments within the body. However, there were four firearm wounds on the surface of the body which indicated the passage of just one bullet through the victim's back, abdomen and left arm. The entry wound was on the right side of the back of the chest, 45 ½ inches above the right heel, 10 inches below the top of the right shoulder, 5 ½ inches to the right of the spine, and 3 ¼ inches behind the back fold of the right armpit. The wound was situated over the position of the 6th and 7th right side ribs.

The entry wound was almost round, measuring seven mm x seven mm and was surrounded by an elliptical rim of abrasion set obliquely upwards and to the right. The rim of the abrasion measured four mm at its upper end and one mm and one and a half mm wide around the lower end and sides of the bullet hole. The bullet track passed downwards, forwards and towards the left, travelling sharply downwards in the tissues of the chest wall at an angle of 60-70 degrees to the horizontal plane of her body. It penetrated the rib cage between the tenth and eleventh ribs in the right side, some two and a half inches below the entry wound on the skin. The bullet track splintered the lower edge of the tenth rib, three inches from the side of the spine. The bullet then passed through the right lobe of the diaphragm, and entered the right lobe of the liver just above the outer extremity of the bare area of the organ. It then penetrated through the right lobe, extensively lacerating it to exit from the liver just below and to the right of the neck of the gallbladder. The exit wound in the right lobe of the

71

liver was three inches in diameter.

The bullet then penetrated the inferior vena cava below the liver and was deflected upwards against the side of the spine, which showed a small area of bruising. The right adrenal gland had been lacerated by the bullet prior to its entry into the vena cava. After deflection, the bullet passed through the head of the pancreas and then re-entered the left lobe of the liver bursting it upwards and outwards. The bullet then left the chest by passing through the left lobe of the diaphragm and notching the lower edge of the left lower costal margin and produced a twelve mm by eight mm exit wound on the front of the lower left chest. This wound was almost rectangular with one rounded end and was surrounded by an almost bullet-shaped rim of abrasion laid obliquely upwards and to the right.

The victim's left elbow appeared to have been held in contact with the side of her left chest, with her elbow bent at right angles at the moment she was shot. The re-entry injury was kidney-shaped and was surrounded by bullet-shaped abrasions mirroring the abrasion surrounding the exit wound on her chest and consistent with the entry of a tumbling bullet. The angle of the bullet wound track indicated that she was shot in the back by a person who was situated at a considerably higher level. Assuming that she was standing upright at the moment she was shot, the track would indicate that she had been shot from one of the adjacent floors of an adjacent building. Again, assuming that she was standing when she was shot, it would have been impossible for the bullet wound to have been caused by a person situated nearby at ground level."

Source: Dr Iain West's Casebook, Chester Stern, (Warner Books, London, 1997, pp. 38-48).

Death By Asphyxiation

The term *asphyxia* is from the Greek meaning 'absence of pulsation', In forensic medicine it is defined as 'interference with oxygenation from any source'. The 'mechanism' of asphyxial deaths is 'the lack of oxygen to the body'. Asphyxia is the principal cause of death in acts of homicide, and can occur as the result of suffocation, smothering, choking and crush trauma.

Suffocation

Death will occur when oxygen in the atmosphere falls below a survivable level, and is replaced by Carbon Dioxide (CO^2). Death will then be the result of asphyxia due to carbon dioxide poisoning. Suffocation is usually associated with a person being confined in a small space with very limited oxygen capacity.

The most common occurrence of death from asphyxiation is in mining disasters where miners become trapped underground. Death can also result from persons being in unventilated places which produce Carbon Monoxide (CO). Carbon dioxide is a natural gas present at a concentration of around 0.3% in the atmosphere. It is often present on industrial sites and in places where explosions or fires have just occurred. Its concentration in the lungs prevents the expulsion of CO^2 from the body, so that respiration is restricted. Concentrations as low as three percent in the atmosphere will cause symptoms to appear; dizziness, headaches and general weakness. Concentrations over 25% are fatal.

Carbon Monoxide (CO) is even more deadly since it will bind to haemoglobin to form the very stable compound *carboxyhaemoglobin*. This essentially means that oxygen can no longer be carried by the blood, since the site on the haemoglobin molecule, is now occupied by the CO. Death by CO poisoning is a common form of suicide. The victim usually places their head in an oven or connects a tube from a car exhaust to the inside of the car and lies down, death following soon afterwards.

One of the post-mortem findings of CO poisoning is the development of a bright red tinting on the skin, which is very similar to the colour changes of the skin due to cyanide poisoning. It is the absence of the distinctive *bitter almonds* smell that distinguishes the two.

Smothering

Death is caused by the accidental or homicidal obstruction of the nose and mouth which prevents respiration. Smothering can occur accidentally in the very young, elderly and intoxicated persons. <u>Homicidal</u> smothering occurs if pressure from an assailant's hand is applied to the nostrils and mouth simultaneously, and at the same time, the assailant applies pressure to the victim's chest, preventing the movement of the diaphragm.

Choking

This is caused by a blockage of the air passage by foreign bodies such as vomit, partly-chewed food or dust. Choking is rarely used as a method of homicide. However, there have been recorded cases where victims have choked on material used as 'gags' over their mouths during the commission of burglary.

Crush-Traumatic Asphyxia

This mode of death is almost always the result of an accidental fall of heavy substance like the collapse of a trench, or being pinned down under some weight. Under these circumstances, the chest is compressed which restricts the movement of the diaphragm preventing respiration.

Another common cause is being crushed in a crowd. This is exactly what occurred in April 1989, at the Hillsborough Football Stadium in Sheffield, during the match between Liverpool and Nottingham Forest for the FA Cup semi-final. 95 Liverpool fans were crushed to death against security fencing. They were pinned against the bars by the sheer weight of the bodies pressing down on them.

Strangulation

Death is caused by a constricting force being applied around the neck, using such articles as a rope or scarf. This article is referred to as a <u>ligature</u> and may have been knotted, tied into a running noose or had the ends crossed over. In cases of homicide, some other person than the victim will need to have pulled the ligature tight in order for strangulation to occur.

Death is by asphyxiation and can be the result of accident, suicide or homicide. Ligature marks usually appear as a furrow or furrows impressed horizontally around the victim's neck. This mark will appear lower than that caused by 'hanging', because the body's weight has not pulled on the noose. It is the nature of the ligature employed, and the degree of pressure on the neck that dictates the physical appearance of the marks. For example, a wire noose would produce a thin deep mark, but that made by a soft material would be hardly noticeable on the skin of the neck.

In cases of suicidal strangulation, this is effected by the victim themselves who tie and tighten the ligature around the neck usually more than once. This is to ensure that constant pressure is maintained when the victim has become unconscious. In any investigation of suspected suicide by strangulation, it is vital that any ligature is photographed at the scene *in situ* while still around the victim's neck.

Manual Strangulation

This is often referred to as <u>throttling</u>, and is caused by compression of the throat by the hands and fingers of an assailant. This can be accomplished single-handed in which the thumb of a right-handed assailant is pressed into the right-hand side of a victim's neck close to the angle of the jaw. The signs of throttling may consist of bruising or superficial abrasion of the neck, corresponding to a number of thumb and finger pads. The signs of death from throttling depend upon the precise mode of death. There are essentially three mechanisms:

1. The windpipe is occluded which results in oxygen deficiency and the presence of 'petechial haemorrhages'.
2. The blood supply is cut off due to pressure applied to the <u>carotid arteries</u>.
3. Death from <u>vagal inhibition</u> of the heart. Any sudden unexpected and partially abnormal sensory stimulation may result in a sudden and abnormal reflex through the motor component of the vagus nerve, resulting in the heart arresting and death occurring with great suddenness.

The <u>carotid plexus</u> in the neck is particularly sensitive,and pressure at this point may well be the predominant cause of this type of sudden death. Also, fracture of the laryngeal cartilages may provide the main reflux stimulus.

Injuries to the tissue and larynx provide the most important findings in the post-mortem dissection after manual strangulation. Bruising is the most constant finding corresponding to the pressure marks under the fingers.

Fracture of the laryngeal cartilages is another common finding. This is because the position of the thumb in manual strangulation rests on the ligament that joins the thyroid cartilage to the hyoid bone which is very often fractured. Damage to the larynx and fracture of the main wings of the thyroid gland will imply considerable force having been used. Also, these types of fractures can result from the Karate style of blow from an assailant rather than simple throttling.

In cases of strangulation by ligature, the main post-mortem findings are those of facial congestion. The ligature mark in the neck is deep and is opposite the point of suspension. It often passes between the hyoid and thyroid cartilages in front, rising to the point of an inverted letter 'V', corresponding to the knot of the noose, either in the midline at the rear or behind an ear.

Death By Drowning

Corpses in water always lie face downwards, with the head hanging. Buffeting in the water often produces post-mortem head injuries. These may be difficult to distinguish from injuries sustained during the life of the victim. The presence of bleeding usually distinguishes ante-mortem from post-mortem injuries. The normal changes of decomposition of a body are delayed in cold,deep water, so that bodies may be well-preserved after a long period of immersion. These conditions are favourable to the formation of 'adipocere' which is 'goose-skin' on the skin, which also protects against decomposition.

When a body is recovered from water, two critical questions arise. Firstly, was the victim alive or dead when he/she entered the water? And secondly, is the cause of death drowning, (or if not, what is the cause of death)?

To resolve these questions, information must be obtained regarding the circumstances preceding the victim's death, the circumstances of recovery of the body, and the findings of the post-mortem examination.

Drowning can be defined as 'suffocation due to immersion of the nostrils and the mouth in a liquid'. The mechanism of death is complex, and not simply asphyxiation due to suffocation. Submersion is followed by struggle which then subsides due to exhaustion, then drowning begins. When the breath can be held no longer, water is inhaled, with associated coughing and vomiting. This is rapidly followed by loss of consciousness and death within minutes.

Drowning results from a combination of the effects of water on the blood, and when air is prevented from entering the air passages and lungs by the water. Although the severity of post-mortem signs of anoxia will depend on how much the victim struggles while in the water, if no signs of anoxia are present, then the cause of death was not drowning, even though the body was recovered from the water. It is not necessary for the body or even the whole head to be submerged, it requires only the mouth and nostrils to be under water for anoxia to result.

The Process of Drowning

In a typical case, the victim will begin to panic from the first ingestion of water into the air passages. In the subsequent struggle, sufficient water will be ingested into the lungs to mix with air and mucus, to produce a choking froth. At the same time the lungs will become water-logged and heavy, making it difficult to remain afloat. Struggling will cease for a short time before a final burst of convulsions will lead ultimately to death.

There is the likelihood that if a person is suddenly and unexpectedly plunged into cold water, cardiac inhibition will cause the condition known as *reflex cardiac arrest*. In this case, signs of drowning will not be present. Such sudden death may also be induced in people who are heavily intoxicated when they enter the water.

Post-Mortem Appearances

There are few external symptoms of drowning, the main one being the fine white foam created by the mixture of air, water and mucus which appears at the nostrils and mouth. Other signs will be a wrinkling of the skin on the palm of the hands and soles of the feet, if the victim has been in the water for any length of time.

In cases of suspected drowning, the pathologist will look for the presence of objects such as stones or water weeds which have been grabbed at during the pre-death struggle, and become locked in the clenched fist by cadaveric spasm, one certain indication of death by drowning. Autopsy will reveal the lungs to be pale and distended, and when the thoracic cavity is opened up, they will tend to 'balloon out'.

The trachea and bronchi will be found to contain foam, together with the lungs when sectioned. Water is usually present in the stomach and oesophagus, and may also contain debris such as weeds and algae. In most cases of drowning, haemorraging will be found in the middle ear, caused by barometric pressure. Tests will be performed to ascertain the presence of any factors which may have contributed to the drowning. These include not only evidence of disease and illness, but the presence of alcohol and drugs.

It has been reported that of domestic drownings in a bath, those resulting from drug overdoses are as highs as 50% of the total (in the UK).

All injuries on the body must be carefully examined by the pathologist and recorded, these do not necessarily indicate homicide. A body in water is subjected to many hazards such as being struck by boats, submerged objects etc.

Diatom Tests

When death is caused by drowning in 'natural' water like lakes, rivers and canals, the water entering the body will contain microscopic organisms called <u>diatoms</u> while the blood is still circulating through the body. These diatoms will be distributed around the body, finding their way into the organs, brain and even bone marrow. If the body is already dead when it enters the water, diatoms will not be present.

The diatom phenomenon is useful in investigating whether the place where the body was recovered was the actual site of death of the victim. Diatoms can be identified with their area of origin with considerable accuracy due to the fact that any combination of species is likely to be unique to a recognised location. Forensic investigations of suspected cases of drowning are a challenge to the forensic pathologist because the mechanism of death in drowning is neither simple or uniform.

Circumstances and Manner of Death in Drowning

The global incidence of death by drowning is estimated at around 5.8 per 100,000 population. Approximately 1,500 deaths from drowning occur in the UK annually, with 25% occurring at sea, the rest in inland waters.

The majority of victims are young adults and children, two-thirds are accidental, one-third suicidal, and homicidal drowning is relatively rare. Accidental drowning of children mainly occur in fish ponds, the bath or swimming pools. Accidental drowning in adults is commonly associated with alcohol consumption, males being predominant. In suicidal drowning, some clothes may be left in a neat pile close to the water, the pockets may be filled with stones or weights tied to the body. The hands or the feet are sometimes tied together, and an examination of the ligatures will show whether they could have been tied by the victim. Persons jumping from a bridge or cliff into water may suffer injuries from impact with rocks or the water itself. In fact, impact with the water can produce severe fatal injuries such as fractures of the ribs, sternum or thoracic spine with lacerations of the heart and lungs.

Homicidal drowning is uncommon and requires either contact between the assailant and the victim, or a victim who is incapacitated by disease, drink or drugs, or taken by surprise. Disposal in water may be attempted where the victim has already been killed by other means.

Autopsy is directed towards establishing injuries that are inconsistent with accident in the absence of the usual signs of drowning. The investigation of a death in a domestic bath is difficult due to the lack of accurate information concerning the position of the body as found, and the level of water in the bath.

First, it must be established whether the nose and mouth were actually under the water. Such drownings will only occur if the victim is unconscious by reason of disease, or the consumption of alcohol or drugs, or has suffered a head injury. Where the victim is a woman of child-bearing age, then pregnancy and abortion should be suspected. Also, the domestic bathroom presents other hazards in addition to drowning – electrocution or carbon monoxide poisoning from faulty heaters, for example. Persons unconscious by reason of natural disease or injury, can drown in quite shallow water, providing it is sufficiently deep to cover the nose and mouth.

Individuals engaged in underwater swimming competitions may hyperventilate prior to entering the water. This can result in sudden loss of consciousness and drowning. The survival rate for potentially fatal <u>salt-water</u> submersion is about 80%, whereas in fresh water, it is less than 50%.

Not all water deaths are necessarily 'drownings'. <u>Vagal inhibition</u> caused by a sudden change in temperature, such as falling into icy water, may cause death before actual drowning takes place. It was often believed that those passengers who died when the *Titanic* sank in 1912, were drowned, when in fact, they died of 'hypothermia'.

The action of the inhalation and swallowing of water during drowning results in massive disturbance to the body's 'osmotic balance'. As a result, drowning in fresh water is usually very rapid. This is because the blood is diluted to such an extent that water will enter the blood's cells causing them to rupture. In sea water, drowning is much slower, because the increase in osmotic pressure in the blood will cause water to flow out of the blood into the plasma.

Head Injuries

Approximately one million patients present to hospital annually in the UK with head injuries. Ninety percent of these are classed as 'mild' or 'minor', five per cent 'moderate' and five per cent 'severe' injuries. Death from head injury in the UK has an incidence of between six and ten per 100,000 population each year.

Head injuries are of particular importance to forensic pathology because the head is often targeted in assaults, and the brain and its coverings are more vulnerable to a degree of trauma that would not reasonably be lethal if applied to other areas of the body.

Blunt force trauma (BFT) is one of the most common injuries encountered by the forensic pathologist in a variety of scenarios. These include jumping or falling from heights, blast injuries and being struck by firm objects. Blunt force injuries located in the skull are often associated with the cause of death. This makes their examination of vital importance in the medico-legal investigation of death.

The first question that emerges in cases of head injury is the timing of injuries, and whether they coincide with the time of death. Forensic pathology uses the terms *ante-mortem* to mean 'before death', *peri-mortem* to mean 'at or around the time of death', and *post-mortem* meaning 'after death', in describing the timing of injuries to the body generally.

However, the term 'post-mortem' has a different meaning within different disciplines. In medico-legal terms, it refers to 'an injury that was provoked around the time of death, and is probably associated with the 'cause of death'.

Head injuries have long been considered as the most common 'mechanical' cause of death in road traffic

83

accident, falls and suicidal jumps from high places.

However, 'blunt force cranial trauma' can also occur as a result of inter- personal violence. In particular, 'depressed fractures of the skull' have a high correlation to personal violent acts. Multiple cranial injuries are more frequently associated with violent events than single injuries.

When a head is either struck with or strikes an object having a broad flat surface area, the skull at the point of impact flattens out to conform to the shape of the surface against which it impacted. Skeletal injuries are often encountered during post-mortem examinations in various occasions, collision accidents, suicidal falls and homicides. When a 'tool' impression is present, a comparison of casts of a suspected tool and its impression can be undertaken.

Also the use of MRI imaging is used in the investigation of blunt force trauma to the skull. Different skulls will have different 'tolerance' to head injuries depending upon the skull's thickness, the age of the individual, and the circumstances surrounding the impact. The average adult skull weighs about four and a half kg, and a 'simple fracture' can occur by just walking into a fixed object.

Based on the direction of the blow, the most inward displaced fragment of bone will be <u>opposite</u> to the direction of the striking object. 'Lines of fracture' are typically longer on the side of the bone opposite to the surface of the impact. <u>Low-speed injuries</u> involving a wide area of the skull typically produce <u>linear fractures,</u> while <u>high-speed</u> trauma results in smaller <u>depressed fractures</u>. Blunt force trauma, with the exclusion of ballistic trauma, is considered to be a 'low-speed' injury.

The response of bone to <u>load</u> or strain depends upon the velocity or speed and weight of the force being applied. A slow-load includes vehicular accidents, falling from heights, aircraft crashes and assaults. Upon slow loading, bone can return to its original shape after the force is removed, deform permanently or fracture. The presence of at least one blunt laceration, one deep contusion and evidence of 'intracranial trauma' are highly indicative of homicide.

'Linear fractures' on the right side of the skull are more prominent in falls. This is because the victim's first response to falls is to try to interpose their right hand, and therefore the right side of the head is more prone to hit the ground. Conversely, left-sided cranial fractures are more frequently associated with blows coming from a right-handed perpetrator.

For the differentiation between 'violent assaults', such as a blow to the head with a blunt instrument, and accidents such as a fall, the *Hat Brim Line* or HBL rule is proposed as a single criterion. The HBL corresponds to the maximum circumference of the vault of the skull. Lesions outside it are more frequently attributed to a blow rather than a fall.

The effectiveness of a blunt instrument depends upon two factors – its weight or mass, and the velocity or speed with which is its delivered. The resulting force of the blow is referred to as its *kinetic energy*, and can be expressed by the following equation:

$$E = \frac{m \times v^2}{2}$$

where E = kinetic energy, m = mass or weight and v = velocity or speed.

This equation clearly demonstrates that the speed in which a weapon is travelling at the time impact is made, has the greater effect because it is 'squared'. This means that a strong blow even with a piece of wood will cause more damage than a weak blow with say a hammer, in general terms. Among the most common 'blunt instruments' are hammers, bats, pokers and even frying pans. Once the head (skull) is cracked with a blow, damage to the brain and its surrounding membranes will occur. *Epidural haematoma* or haemorrhaging (bleeding outside the *dura mater,* the tough membrane lining the skull) can occur due to the tearing of the blood vessels supplying the brain. This type of injury is most common among teenagers. The blood accumulates between the 'dura' and the base of the skull. Quite often, there is no external injury evident apart from bruising to the skin at the site of impact. However, in reality, the accumulation of blood internally puts pressure on the brain itself.

This can result in death within a few hours, due to a blood clot formed at the site of the bleeding, classed as *cerebral haemorrhage.* Subarachnoid haemorrhages are often caused by natural events such as a blow to the head in sporting activities. These are generally associated with 'aneurysms' where the arteries dilate due to weakness in the arterial wall, leading to a balloon-like swelling. Sometimes even a light blow can cause haemorrhaging.

However, at post-mortem, bleeding without an aneurysm raises cause for concern. Blows to the head even with a fist, can cause damage to the brain, due to movement of the brain itself within the skull cavity. The blow in itself may not cause damage, but if the head twists round at some speed as a result of the blow, the brain will be chafed against the inside of the skull, since it is travelling faster than the skull.

Another type of head injury is known as *contre-coup.* This results when the skull strikes the ground after a fall. The resultant injury occurs at a site opposite to that at which the head impacted. For example, if someone falls backwards as in a slipping accident, striking the back of their head on the ground, injury will be to the front of the brain. This is because the skull is travelling much faster than the brain which will receive chafing injuries to the 'frontal and temporal lobes'. A child's skull will bend before breaking, but since blood vessels will be torn in the

86

process, head injury in children often shows a surprising amount of haemorrhaging when compared with the relative lack of damage inflicted to the skull. It is usual for lines of stress fracture to radiate from the point of contact, while the part of the skull struck is depressed. These are referred to as 'lineal' and 'depressed' fractures. This situation is almost exactly comparable with striking the shell of a hard-boiled egg. These radiating fractures may damage blood vessels over a wide area. This explains why death results from what appear to be relatively mild impact injuries.

The membranes of the brain, together with their blood vessels, may be crushed or torn beneath a depressed fracture. More seriously, the brain itself may be lacerated either by the instrument causing the external injury, or by the fragments of bone that are forced inwards by the impact. These are characteristic of homicidal head injuries.

Following a blunt force head injury, there may be loss of consciousness. In general, the <u>longer</u> the period of unconsciousness and the <u>deeper</u> the coma, the more likely it is that irrecoverable brain damage has occurred. *Cerebral concussion* or stunning following head injury is characterised by temporary loss of consciousness. This is due to a disturbance of brain function without any identifiable pathological changes in the brain itself. This is commonly seen in an individual who has suffered a minor head injury from, say, punches to the head. Concussion may be followed in survivors by *retrograde amnesia*, which is loss of memory extending backwards in time from the moment of impact.

In clinical practice, the severity of a head injury is assessed using the <u>Glasgow Coma Scale</u> (GCS) which produces a numerical score from three being the worst, to fifteen indicating normal responses. This is based upon the assessment of three areas of response; ocular, verbal and motor response. When the brain is damaged following head injury, it may be the immediate result of the physical force, known as <u>primary trauma</u>. This encompasses blunt force trauma to the scalp, skull fracture, lacerations to the brain and inter-cranial haemorrhages. <u>Secondary trauma</u> includes hypoxia, brain swelling resulting in raised inter-cranial pressure and infection. Such infection is usually the consequence of a skull fracture which allows bacteria to enter the subarachnoid space, resulting in *meningitis.*

Blunt force injuries to the scalp particularly abrasions, are indicative of the point of impact. Bruising of the scalp is associated with prominent tissue swelling if the survival time is sufficiently long enough for this to develop. Since the scalp is <u>very vascular</u>, any lacerations bleed profusely, leaving <u>blood spatter</u> evidence at the scene of an attack. Any blunt weapon producing a scalp injury may have <u>trace evidence</u> in the form of blood, tissue and hair present on it. For comparison purposes, a control hair sample and a DNA sample will be routinely taken from the victim.

A skull fracture is an indicator of the application of a significant degree of force to the head, with the associated risk of intra-cranial haemorrhage and cerebral injuries. It is the associated intra-cranial trauma, rather than the skull fracture itself, which is life-threatening.

When blunt force is applied to the skull, some distortions in shape can occur. Forces are transmitted along the bony buttresses towards the skull base until the structure yields, resulting in a fracture at the point of <u>maximum stress</u>. This is commonly distant from the point of impact on the head. The force required to cause a fracture is very variable. It can result from merely walking into a fixed obstruction, falling on to a hard surface, running into an obstruction or from an object thrown with moderate force. In cases where a victim is typically intoxicated, with poor co-ordination, and lack of control of head movements, this can result in a head impact. This is most commonly the result of a punch or sometimes a kick. Occasionally, this can be a fall following a punch or a push. This will result in immediate unconsciousness and death within minutes and without any recovery of consciousness. In such a scenario, the fatal outcome is commonly a complete surprise to the perpetrator and any witnesses.

The point of impact to the head may be anywhere on its circumference. It is the accompanying underlying circumstances that contribute to the final outcome. In some individuals who die within minutes of a head injury, the only post-mortem findings within the brain, will be pin-point haemorrhages in the white matter of the frontal and temporal lobes. It is for the forensic pathologist to determine whether the impact was the result of a fall or a blow to the head. This can reduce a charge of murder to one of manslaughter.

Injuries and Death on Roads

Road traffic incidents comprise a leading cause of injury and death globally. Investigations of vehicular incidents provide important information not only for the investigation of criminal or civil legal proceedings, but also for the development of preventative measures. The overall purpose of accident investigation is to reconstruct the sequence of events leading to a crash. This involves an evaluation of the vehicles involved, the road, the environment and human factors.

The documentation and evaluation of the first three elements is the province of the police road traffic investigator. The evaluation of the human factors is the area of the forensic pathologist. This involves the interpretation of alcohol and drug levels, and in particular, the patterns of injury sustained by those involved.

Pedestrians

In frontal impacts of a vehicle on a pedestrian, five patterns are recognisable. The first of these is known as the wrap pattern, in which the pedestrian is struck by the vehicle's bumper and by the front edge of the bonnet. This causes the body to rotate so that the head, shoulders and chest strike the bonnet and windscreen. This pattern will result in injuries to the lower leg, upper leg or pelvis, the head and chest.

If at the car was braking at the time of the impact,it causes the victim to come off the front and slide across the road surface. In the 'wrap' pattern, the distance between the initial point of impact, and the point on the road surface where the victim strikes the ground, is known as the throw distance. This distance can be correlated with the speed of the vehicle, provided that the vehicle was braking hard immediately after the impact.

The second pattern is called the forward projection. This occurs with high-fronted vehicles or when a small child is struck by car. Following the 'primary impact', the victim is thrown forward onto the road surface with the risk of over-running by any following vehicles.

The third pattern is known as wing top which occurs when the pedestrian is struck by the front wing of the vehicle, being carried over the wing and falling to the ground at the side of the vehicle.

The fourth pattern known as the roof-top pattern occurs only at high speeds or if the vehicle accelerates after impact with the pedestrian. This causes the victim to slide up the front of the vehicle, over the roof to fall on the road behind the vehicle.

The fifth pattern known as the somersault pattern occurs in a high speed impact, when there is sufficient force at the primary impact to somersault the victim into the air. In such cases, there is no secondary impact between pedestrian and vehicle, the victim impacts with the road surface.

The typical pedestrian struck by a vehicle is in an upright position, the primary impact being between the vehicle bumper or fender and the pedestrian's legs. Damage to the bumper, lights and front of the vehicle will reflect the point of the primary impact. Abrasion and patterned bruise/abrasions will impact the shape of the component of the vehicle or clothing crushed between the vehicle, and the victim's skin will indicate the point of impact.

If a pedestrian is struck side-on, then this may be obvious from the injury to the side of one leg. The level of impact above the heel, measured with the victim still wearing footwear, can be compared with the ground to bumper height of the vehicle, as well as the injury pattern to the pedestrian.

The height of the bumper does vary between vehicles. However, European cars average between sixteen and twenty inches (40-50 cm) above the ground. This will correspond to the level of the 'upper tibia' of a pedestrian. This also implies that the foot was fixed on the ground at the moment of impact. Since the primary impact is below the centre of gravity of an adult's body, the pedestrian is thrown up onto the front of the vehicle to strike the bonnet and windscreen with resultant secondary impact injuries.

Severe head injuries may occur at this time with associated damage to the vehicle and trace evidence from the vehicle present in the wounds. At the same time, blood, tissue and hair are deposited on the vehicle.

If a pedestrian is struck from behind, the backward arching of the body may cause multiple stretch lacerations in the groin and lower abdomen. In this case, a pedestrian will be over-run rather than thrown onto the bonnet if the vehicle is high-fronted such as a bus, truck or van. If the pedestrian is a small adult or child, they will be struck above the centre of gravity.

In the typical situation with a pedestrian receiving primary impact injuries from the bumper, and secondary impact injuries from being thrown onto the vehicle, the victim then strikes the ground to sustain <u>tertiary</u> impact injuries, commonly to the head and torso. Abrasions associated with these injuries commonly have traces of the roadway surface embedded in them.

In broad grazed abrasions, the multiple levels of accentuation indicate the direction of movement. One clearly delineated end to such an abrasion indicates the start, the initial contact with the roadway, and the other poorly delineated end indicates the finish of the moving contact on the ground. The overall severity of pedestrian injury increases in proportion to the <u>weight and speed</u> of the vehicle.

For any given impact, the elderly will sustain more numerous and severe injuries. When a pedestrian is over-run by a second vehicle following after the one which first struck the pedestrian, then the over-running injuries, although severe, may show minimal haemorrhage because the victim may already be dead.

Vehicular Occupants

The pattern and severity of injuries sustained by vehicle occupants during a collision is influenced by the <u>force</u> of the impact, and its direction, as well as any intrusion into the passenger compartment. The location of the person within the vehicle, the use of seatbelts and the deployment of air-bags are other factors that require consideration.

The most important factor is the rate of <u>deceleration</u> of the vehicle. Spreading the deceleration over a longer time period through the crash design of the vehicle, facilitates a steady deformation of the vehicle's frame. Injuries to vehicle passengers are produced by impact with the interior of the vehicle, <u>distortion</u> of the vehicle frame which intrudes into the interior, and partial or complete <u>ejection</u> of the passenger from the vehicle. Wearing a seatbelt substantially reduces the risk of ejection, but it does not eliminate it completely. Intrusion into the passenger compartment is more likely in <u>high-speed</u> collisions. Vehicle roll-overs increase the risk of severe and fatal injuries. If vehicle occupants are <u>unrestrained</u>, then roll-over crashes are commonly fatal as the result of partial or complete ejection from the vehicle.

Side impacts can produce severe injuries because the vehicle side provides poor protection against intrusion. Side impacts generally produce more severe injuries than frontal impacts even in restrained occupants because the seatbelts are less effective. Seatbelts and air-bags may protect against impact with the interior of the vehicle but cannot protect from severe deceleration forces in high-speed collisions.

The classically-described injuries of vehicle occupants are those occurring in a head-on collision, <u>without</u> the use of safety restraints. In these situations, at impact, forward movement of the driver and front-seat passenger produces <u>knee</u> impact against the fascia with soft tissue injuries and possible fractures. Bracing for impact, by pressing the feet against the floor, results in lower leg injuries to the passenger, while hard braking may cause a similar injury to one leg of the driver. Continued upward and forward movement of the occupants produces head impact against the roof interior and windscreen, and chest impact against the steering wheel, or in the case of the front passenger, the dashboard.

Unrestrained rear seat passengers will sustain lower leg injuries, and head and torso injuries from striking the back of the front seat, together with chest injuries which almost always include rib fractures.

Seat Belts and Air-Bags

A seatbelt prevents ejection from the vehicle and also restrains the body during deceleration, thus protecting the body during deceleration, and protecting the head by preventing impact with the vehicle interior.

However, seatbelts produce their own pattern of internal injuries. A two-point lap belt compresses abdominal organs against the vertebral column and allows hyper-flexion of the body around the seatbelt. Overall, the use of seatbelts, while reducing the severity of injuries, has influenced a pattern of injuries with an increase in facial and skull fractures in drivers, and an increase in rib and sternal fractures and abdominal bruising in vehicle occupants.

Air-bags offer added protection in a collision but are also associated with some risks. Air-bags function by sensing the slowing of a vehicle following impact and detonating an explosive which produces a large volume of gas to fill and deploy the bag. The explosion produces a large amount of white smoke which may be mistaken for a vehicle fire. When the explosive propellant is ignited, the air-bag explodes towards the vehicle occupant at a speed of up to 200 mph.

Injuries can result from contact with either the air-bag cover or the bag itself. The air-bag covers are located in the steering wheel and the dashboard panel on the passenger side. Injuries to the hands and arms (including fractures) are common if either the driver or the front seat passenger makes contact with the air-bag module cover.

Identifying the Driver

Occasionally, when there is a dispute about who was driving and who was a passenger, the injury pattern may help to distinguish. The rapid deceleration of a vehicle crash causes the vehicle occupants, whether restrained or not, to move initially towards the main area of impact. This occupant movement predicts the direction of movement of each occupant, and consequently, what part of the vehicle's interior they will strike, and the type of injury they will sustain. Matching the pattern of injuries to both survivors and those killed, with the interior surfaces and components of the vehicle, helps to identify an occupant's position, and this establishes who was driving the vehicle at the time of the collision.

The classical injury seen in an unrestrained driver is an impact bruise-abrasion on the chest, with underlying fracture of the sternum and ribs, from impact with the steering wheel. However, restrained drivers in frontal impacts typically sustain head injuries due to contact with the steering wheel. Often imprint abrasion against interior fittings can be matched with the causative object and assist in locating the individual within the vehicle at the moment of impact.

Motorcyclists and Cyclists

Motorcyclists commonly sustain leg injuries from the primary impact, but these injuries are rarely fatal. Head and neck injuries resulting from being thrown forward are a common cause of death. The wearing of a helmet will protect against scalp injuries and fractures of the skull, but not against acceleration/deceleration brain injury. The crash helmet should always be examined for evidence of external damage.

A motorcyclist thrown forward and striking the top of his head on the roadway, or other fixed object, may sustain a 'ring-fracture' at the base of the skull when the head is compacted onto the torso. Being thrown off the motorcycle at speed, and sliding along the roadway produces broad patches of prominent grazing abrasions, contaminated with road surface debris known as 'road rash', especially if there is insufficient protection from clothing.

Cyclists are most commonly killed and injured when struck by a motor vehicle, or by a protruding part of a vehicle whilst overtaking. Damage to the cycle rather than to the cyclist may reflect the primary impact, and have trace evidence from the striking vehicle. Cyclists struck from behind often show primary impact bruises or abrasions or both to the area of the buttock and back of the thigh. Secondary impact injuries may result from either being thrown up onto the vehicle or from being knocked to one side onto the roadway.

As with pedestrians, bicyclists may be over-run by succeeding vehicles following the initial collision.

Manner of Death

Not all deaths on the road are accidents. Some are the result of <u>natural disease</u>, and others are suicides or homicides. Natural disease causing sudden death in the driver of a motor vehicle is typically not so rapid in its onset that the driver cannot exercise some control, by slowing the vehicle and veering off the road. When witnessed, the unusual nature of the incident raises the suspicion of natural disease, and typically the vehicle driver has minimal non-lethal injuries which are insufficient to account for death.

Ischaemic heart disease is the main cause of natural death at the wheel, and occasionally the cause can be a disease of the brain. Suicide by motor vehicle represents a very small percent of driver fatalities. Typically, the single occupant will, for no apparent reason, drive the car at high speed into oncoming traffic, often heavy goods vehicles. A driver may use a vehicle as a weapon, deliberately striking a pedestrian, cyclist or other road user. However, this is a very a rare form of homicide.

Chapter Five: Case Studies

Asphyxiation Case

How do you tell the difference between hanging and a murder made to look like a suicide by hanging? Suicides by hanging create a 'signature' pattern of marks around the neck, usually like an inverted 'V' on the back of the neck from the rope's suspension. The pressure of the rope often causes *petechiae*, tiny broken blood vessels which appear as red dots on the face, eyelids and mouth lining.

In contrast, a homicide by strangulation would produce different marks, a straight line across the back of the neck caused by the material used to cut off the air supply, a garrotte made from a belt or cord. Often the perpetrator will leave bruises and contusion around the neck. The attack may also damage internal neck structure, particularly the <u>hyoid bone</u>.

Forensic pathologists use the autopsy or post-mortem examination as a vehicle to determine three facets of a case; the physiological reason for death or <u>mechanism</u> of death, the <u>agent</u> or cause of death, perhaps a gun, knife or rope, and the <u>manner</u> in which the deceased died, say suicide, homicide, natural causes, accident or undetermined.

Sexual Asphyxiation

This is a type of sexual behaviour with an ironical twist; those who indulge in sexual asphyxiation find the sensation of suffocation sexually stimulating, usually accompanied by sexual acts such as masturbation. Asphyxiation is achieved with a plastic bag, chemicals, a partner's hands or most commonly, a noose from a rope, a tie or a sheet. This practice may occur as <u>auto-erotic</u>

98

behaviour which is defined as sexual activity occurring while one is alive, or as a sexual act in which one partner assists in the suffocation or strangulation, using a plastic bag or a garrotte on his or her partner.

In either case, death sometimes results from miscalculation. During auto-erotic sexual asphyxia, the subject often leaves themselves a 'safety release', but if they pass out before they can release the 'choke-hold', asphyxia results. Auto-erotic asphyxia as a sex game is not new. The dynamic is quite simple, one applies pressure to the *carotid artery* with anything from a rope to a belt or chain, and a feeling of fainting results. When the pressure is released, the blood rushes back to the head causing a euphoric feeling or light headedness lasting for a few seconds.

How does the pathologist differentiate between suicide and accident in such a death? Did the victim leave a note or make overtures towards suicide? Is the victim wearing few or no clothes? Is there any evidence of masturbation or ejaculation? Is there a mirror and/or pornographic material at the scene? Did the deceased prepare any devices as safeguards? Does any evidence or history suggest that the victim regularly engaged in sexual asphyxiation?

The presence of a second person makes a significant difference in determining the manner of death. The pathologist cannot rule the subsequent death as a suicide or natural death, because, although unintentional, a person caused the accident, which may place the death in the category of a suspicious death or even murder.

The key elements in the post-mortem of a victim of asphyxiation are the neck structures. The first item to be examined is the hyoid bone that is located in the throat structure. The hyoid structure is the only bone in the human body not touching other bones, and consists of three fused portions that together form a horseshoe.

The hyoid bone provides the pathologist with a vital piece of evidence in making a final determination as to the cause of death. In a murder by strangulation, fractures of the hyoid usually occur at the end of the bones forming the sides of the horseshoe, called the cornua. The constricting neck structures exert pressure on the ends of the hyoid structure and fractures sometimes result, especially in older victims.

Hanging with bed-sheets would not usually cause a fracture of the hyoid. Finding a fracture of the hyoid bone in a hanging, would call into question the suicide manner, and suggest homicide, because the pressure required to fracture the hyoid bone would not likely occur in a suicide where the victim hanged him or herself with a sheet.

Head Trauma

The victim was a 25-year-old male, six feet tall and weighing 235 pounds. The previous evening he was out parting with friends. The party ended with him falling in the bathroom resulting in a blunt-force trauma to the victim's head. He was found unconscious by his friends on the bathroom floor and was taken to the local hospital A&E department. Subsequent blood tests revealed the presence of alcohol and drugs in his system.

With the aid of smelling salts he came round but his speech was incoherent. It was suspected that he had suffered a closed-head injury. The attending doctor administered the Glasgow Coma Scale (GCS) procedure for patients with suspected closed-head injury. His score was nine out of total of fifteen, which confirmed that he probably had a closed-head injury, and he was sent for a CT scan to assess the potential damage.

Thirty to forty minutes later, the physician repeated the GCS tests and obtained a total score of just three. This meant that he did not respond to any type of stimuli, the lowest scale obtainable. This indicated that he did not open his eyes, and had no verbal or motor response, and shortly afterwards he died.

Since this patient died of a head wound, one might think that an examination of only the head and brain was needed to determine the cause and type of head injury. However, a complete post-mortem examination is always performed.

In this case, a dissection of the internal organs revealed no significant disease or defect. Although the dissection on the internal organs is routine procedure, this death is not devoid of mystery. The circumstances in which he was found, and the victim's alleged accident occurring without witnesses created the need for a post-mortem. Did he sustain his fatal head wound as the result of a fall? Did someone hit him during an assault? Did his death result from a cerebral aneurysm?

On removal, the victim's brain was found to be 'soft', resulting from decomposition caused when the body exists at body temperature at 98.6 degrees F for several hours without an oxygen supply to the brain. This patient most likely died from compression and herniation of the brain stem. When a person hits their head, the momentum continues to move the brain, causing it to collide with the skull. This collision causes bruising and swelling to the brain. As a result, the brain would exhibit a certain pattern of bruising which provide tell-tale signs.

The brain stem sits inside a funnel-shaped hole in the base of the skull, the *foramen magnum*. Swelling in the brain stem forces it into a cavity, compressing and subsequently preventing it from functioning properly. The heart is thus kept beating and pumping blood, which in turn denies the brain its supply of oxygen. Without blood supplying oxygen to the brain tissues, death is imminent.

In such cases, doctor have what is referred to in medical practice as the 'golden hour' in which to diagnose and set to work treatments that might reverse this process. Part of the treatment would include evacuating a blood clot from the skull usually via a hole or two, and administering medicine to keep the brain from swelling.

Unfortunately, at this point when this patient hit his head, grains of sand began to fall from a 'golden hourglass'. Forty-five minutes after he arrived at the hospital, the last grain fell, indicating that nature had conquered human effort.

The underside of the patient's skull showed the presence of a fracture. This is the last link in a chain of evidence that negates homicide. A hairline fracture, like a line drawn with a pencil, extending for about one inch about midway up the back of the skull was discovered.

It is hard to believe that a force of 235 pounds striking the rim of a bath tub or a tiled floor would not have done more damage than this fracture. However, the existing skull damage fits the theory that this patient fell and hit the back of his head, sustaining what would become a fatal blow.

An assault would be less likely to leave a linear fracture and, in many cases, would result in depressed fractures, which on the inside of the skull would look like an inverted pock-mark. If someone for example, had hit the patient on the back of the head with a hammer, the hammer would leave a depressed fracture. With wounds caused by such excessively hard blows, fractures would extent or radiate from the depression. Blunt-force trauma to the head can also leave superficial evidence that might appear on examination.

The victim's eyes can also provide evidence. Several blows to the head can cause bleeding inside the skull, *subdural haematoma*. As a result of the compression to the brain, the pupil of the eye on the side of the haemorrhage, will dilate (widen), a condition often referred to as a '<u>blown-pupil</u>'. Thus, 'blown pupils' are the dilated pupils that follow severe blows to the head. Since blown pupils can occur with many types of head trauma, their presence only suggests that the victim sustained some type of head wound, not what type it may be. So this type of fracture is the key piece of forensic evidence in determining what type of blow the victim sustained and the subsequent cause of death.

An actual fall would have likely resulted in this 'linear' crack running a more or less straight vertical line along the back of the victim's skull, which is not the case with a blow from an object such as a hammer or lead pipe.

In this case, the question remained; on what did the victim strike his head? Sustaining a fatal injury in the bathroom may at first seem unlikely, but on consideration, the bathroom does present a prime location for an accident to occur. The typical bathroom offers a number of hard edges on which a person who loses consciousness could strike his or her head; the edges of the sink, the edge of the bathtub itself, plumbing fixtures in the tub, the toilet seat, water cistern etc.

In this particular case, the brain was too soft to dissect at post-mortem. After one week of submersion in formaldehyde, the brain will solidify and be ready for dissection. After eventually dissecting the brain, the pattern of bruising expected from an accidental fall was confirmed. The cause of death in this case was recorded as <u>accidental</u>.

Stabbing Case

The victim was a 22-year-old male who had attended a party the previous evening during, at which an argument ensued between himself and a friend. The victim had become involved with his friend's girlfriend, and during the course of the evening, and after the consumption of drink, the affair was exposed. After a few punches, the two men were separated but their fighting continued in the car park. An eye witness who saw the incident from a distance, reported seeing the perpetrator striking the victim several times with a knife in the chest area, causing the victim to slump and fall to the ground.

The alleged perpetrator, once in police custody, claimed self-defence. This plea failed when considering the victim was unarmed and sustained four knife wounds which proved fatal. He died the same night in hospital.

Like many corpses that appear in the mortuary, the combination of blood and gravity (lividity) creates a bruised appearance to the victim's back. Also, he bears the brand of hospital personnel who attempted in vain to save his life; a few square ECG pads used in an attempt to 'kick-start' his heart, and a chest drain protruding from his left side, inserted to drain blood in his chest cavity caused by the four stab wounds on his torso and hip.

The knife found at the scene, is called a 'butterfly' knife and is available at most surplus and martial arts shops. Several stab wounds perforated the chest; three of them looked like 10p coins with slits at their centres. They looked much too small to have been inflicted by the 'butterfly' knife. They looked more like the products of a thin, narrow blade like a stiletto. The fourth wound in the victim's upper left side, was an inch-long slit that looked like that of the 'butterfly' knife.

The victim sustained three wounds to the chest, one directly under the sternum (breast bone) and two either side of the rib cage. The fourth was on the left upper thigh just below the hip.

The procedure for stabbing victims requires x-rays to determine if a portion of the blade broke off and became lodged inside the wound. A diagram of the male thoracic/abdominal areas, anterior and posterior views, is used to indicate the placement of the four stab wounds. This extends from the neck to the top of the buttocks. After measurements have been taken, the process of examining and investigating the stab wounds begins, with a determination of each wound's 'clock position'.

This is a metaphor adopted by pathologists specifically to describe knife wounds. The elastic fibres in skin deform the wound, causing it to stretch, elongate and pull back around the wound, forming the pale pink circles, the 'clock' that appears around three of the four knife penetrations. The stab wounds are evident inside the reddish interior of the circles, appearing as slits which represent the 'hands' or the original wounds, the ends of the stab wounds point to two different 'clock positions'. One stab wound on the victim's chest points to ten, the other end points to four, giving a 'clock position' of 10:4.

The red tissue inside the circles is muscle. When a knife blade penetrates muscle, the muscle 'grabs' the blade, literally squeezing it. Inserting a knife always meets less resistance than removing it, a fact that explains why the slits appear smaller than they should given the width of the knife that caused the injuries. Knives most often have a dull end and a sharp end.

Wound number three, just to the left of the victim's left nipple inside the circle found by retracted skin, the 'clock face' is the mark left where the knife penetrated the deep reddish/orange muscle, the two edges of the butterfly knife that killed him, the dull end and the sharp end forming a wedge-shaped slit in the reddish/orange muscle.

Wound number four in the victim's upper left thigh, inside the 'clock-face', is a wider less pronounced slit which indicates that the perpetrator twisted the knife handle while the blade was embedded in his victim's thigh. The pathologist uses a probe, which is a long thin blade to determine the path of the knife blade as it penetrated the victim's body, and the depth of each penetration. Wound number two just under the victim's sternum, is likely to have struck the heart.

The legal system requires painstaking procedure for

murder victims because the evidence collected at post-mortem examinations must withstand scrutiny in court. A significant portion of medico-legal post-mortems on murder victims, consist of describing and investigating wounds and other evidence, such as the victim's clothing worn at the time of the crime.

The wound to the victim's upper left thigh appeared very deep. The probe revealed that the butterfly knife penetrated five inches into the hip, which does suggest that the blade could have nicked the <u>femoral artery</u> which could lead to a fatal loss of blood within minutes. When the case comes to court, the prosecution will most likely show the jury the murder weapon, the butterfly knife, and when they are told that the victim's killer sank the blade five inches into his upper thigh, they will realise that this means he sank the knife blade to the hilt, a vivid depiction of the ferocity of the crime.

The last shirt worn by the victim, a blue t-shirt is covered with streaks of still wet coagulating blood. This t-shirt is studied very carefully, probing the holes caused by the knife wounds, identifying the holes, and matching the evidence on the clothes with that on the body. This enables a correspondence between the holes in the shirt and the stab wounds one, two and three. During the post-mortem, the final wound is sought; the depth of the wound and any other evidence of natural disease. It was obvious in this case that the knife wounds killed the victim. However, if some natural disease is found, relatives can be warned in case they may be afflicted with the same predisposition for the disease.

There are various facial wounds, bruises and contusions, evidence suggesting the deceased engaged in a frenzied fight prior to his death. In the fight, the victim sustained four knife wounds, one or two of which pierced his heart, causing a flood of blood into the <u>pericardial sac</u>. His compressed heart stopped beating and he died. Within minutes of the fatal wound, he slumped to the ground according to the eyewitness.

The surfaces of the heart and lungs indicated that the knife wounding the side of the left nipple pierced the edge of the lung and the left ventricle of the heart. The path of the wound under the sternum, three and a half inches long, penetrated the heart causing significant damage. This wound proved fatal and lead to compression of the heart, killing the victim.

Suicide – Carbon Monoxide Poisoning

A 56-year-old male went to bed at midnight in the guest room which he sometimes did. He placed a pillow in the bed to make it appear occupied, to prevent his wife from discovering his preconceived plan. Sometime during the course of the night, his wife checked on the victim and discovered his ruse. However, by then he had completed his intended act in his garage, where she found him outside his car, having committed suicide.

Crime scene investigators found the front seat of his car made into a makeshift bed, a garden hose channelling noxious exhaust fumes into the car, the keys in the ignition in the 'on' position. The carbon monoxide may have left him disorientated and nauseous so he came outside of the car. Another possibility exists; someone else killed him and altered the scene to make it appear to be a suicide. However, this would be an extremely unlikely scenario because the man left a suicide note citing his failing health, and suggesting that his wife would be better off without him.

The victim suffered from bipolar disorder, a chemical imbalance that causes alternating swings between deep depression and intense mania. Six months previously, he tried to kill his wife with a pistol that he had planned to then use on himself in a botched attempt to end both of

107

their lives. According to his wife, he had formulated a supernatural explanation for the pains that troubled him; he believed that demons haunted him.

On examination of the victim's body, a large purple abrasion was found at the base of his spine. More scrapes appeared under the left arm. Sometimes with carbon monoxide poisoning, the victim experiences convulsions which perhaps accounted for these wounds. The wife did find him sprawled out on the concrete floor in their garage.

A toxicology screening test of the victim's blood determined a significant amount of carbon monoxide within his blood. The post-mortem examination, a massive skull fracture was discovered which then called into question the determination of death by suicide. The muscle under the chest wall revealed a 'cherry red' colouration

This is caused by carbon monoxide in the blood. Dissection of the heart revealed atherosclerosis. This occurs when the lumen or walls of the coronary arteries narrow and decrease the flow of blood, resulting in a build-up of fatty deposits called plaque. The coronary arteries in this victim had thickened, hardened and calcified. The victim also suffered from emphysema, which was revealed on examination of his lungs.

His internal organs formed a picture of poor health, created by damaging life-style choices. Charcoal black blotches called 'anthracotic' pigment due to deposition of carbon particles from cigarette smoking, covered the outside of his lungs (the visceral pleura). The inside of the lung tissue was dotted with bullae or holes in the lining walls from years of smoke damage. The lungs function much like a filter and tiny alveoli, millions of them in each lung, stretch and expand with each breath of air, passing oxygen in air into the bloodstream. With each exhalation, the alveoli contract, sending the remainder in the form of carbon dioxide out of the body.

Emphysema destroys alveoli and causes the

surviving ones to lose their elasticity, upon exhalation, they over-expand and never fully contract, trapping air. Consequently, breathing becomes progressively harder. Smoking causes the majority of emphysema cases. Inhalation of smoke destroys the delicate hairs called 'cilia' that cover the bronchial passages and block bacteria, fungi and other harmful substances from entering the lungs. Without the protective cilia, germs invade the lungs and cause pneumonia.

At first, the victim would have experienced trouble catching his breath after physical activity, eventually walking up a flight of stairs would have left him 'gasping' for breath. A persistent and ever-present cough or hack would have accompanied him. He would have felt a constant exhaustion and experienced a loss of appetite and subsequent loss of weight. It appeared that this victim suffered from a number of physical ailments, and in his later years lived a life tinged by discomfort and pain, which, in conjunction with his bipolarism, provided a motive for suicide.

Cardiac Failure and Head Trauma

The victim, a male found in the afternoon lying feet first on the floor of his home, was last seen alive at 8:00 am, having complained of chest pains. Although his heart had stopped beating sometime in the interval, the emergency response team administered a cocktail of drugs, including atropine and adrenaline.

On arrival at the hospital, a heart defibrillator was used, but after three minutes had elapsed, there was no response, no blood pressure and no pulse. After a further two minutes, the heart monitor gave a warning siren as a flat line ran across the screen. The attending physician pronounced the 56-year old victim dead.

The victim's case history contained a list of physical

109

problems he suffered before his fatal collapse. In addition to hypertension, he suffered from diabetes.

Police investigators quoted neighbours describing him as a contentious man with many enemies. Many enemies make many suspects, each with a motive should the post-mortem provide evidence that the cause of death was homicide.

Since the victim probably died of a fatal cardiac arrhythmia, and his case history of hypertension would support this possibility, the heart will most likely provide the key clues to the ultimate cause of death in this case.

At the post-mortem, the liver appeared as a <u>yellow mass</u> in the upper right quadrant of the victim's torso cavity; a certain sign of alcohol abuse. Excessive intake of alcohol can cause 'fatty change' in the liver, the fat accumulation within the cells damage, then change the colour of the liver from its normal dark brown to a golden yellow colour. However, the victim's diabetes could have affected the liver in a similar way.

The appearance of his lungs suggested that the victim also enjoyed smoking. Small black dots tattooing the skin of the lungs were present. The carbon or black patches on lungs do not alone indicate that the victim suffered from emphysema. Coal miner's lungs would blacken from inhalation of coal particles while working in the mine, but they would experience no ill effects, and their lungs would function as normal unless they also smoked. The presence of mucus in the victim's lungs is evidence that he suffered from <u>bronchitis</u>.

Smoking impedes the normal functioning of the lungs, it damages the bronchial glands that produce mucus. The mucus represents a manifestation of the bronchitis and often causes in long-term smokers, a 'wet cough'. The inside of the lungs showed more damage done by years of smoking. The interior of the lungs had mottled appearance of alternating black and crimson blotches. By spraying a steam of water on the surfaces of the lungs, small sponge-like holes could be seen. The holes called *bullae*, result from damage to the minute spaces in the lung where oxygen is absorbed into, and carbon dioxide excreted from the blood.

During the dissection of the heart, small incisions were made through each coronary artery to determine the degree of narrowing. An examination of the victim's coronary arteries revealed that the most severe narrowing was about 20%. As a general rule, 75% of coronary artery must be blocked in order to cause a fatal cardiac arrhythmia.

This patient died when his heart stopped, but what caused his heart to stop? He could have died from the effects of diabetes. The *vitreous humur,* the fluid in the eyes, is examined, for if he died from the effects of diabetes, the eye fluid would contain chemical proof. Then again, he could have overdosed on alcohol or drugs, which would appear in a toxicology report. The diabetes could have caused the yellow discolouration of the liver. If caused by diabetes though, damage to the kidneys would also occur, and no such damage was revealed from a close examination of the kidneys.

Instead of the usual off-white colour of the brain, the entire left frontal portion appeared as a thick reddish brain mass representing a massive bleeding, a *sub-dural haematoma.*

This bleeding indicated the dynamic that caused the victim's heart to stop, but also raised the question as to what caused the head injury in the first place? If he died of a head wound, what caused it? Did he suffer from a brain aneurysm or did he fall and strike his head? Did someone strike him? Would this heart attack victim also become a murder victim?

If someone hit him in the head, most likely but not always, some damage would appear on the outside of the head. Upon close examination of the scalp, there was no superficial damage revealed. While a blow to the head with an object like a hammer would leave a depressed fracture that radiating outwards from a point of impact, very much like a chip in a car windscreen, a blow from a larger blunt instrument with a large surface area such as a board may leave the scalp and skull undamaged.

There was no skull fracture evident but this in itself did not not preclude a blow to the head. The victim had a thick skull so a blow with a blunt object could have caused the internal bleeding, but not a skull fracture. Regardless of what caused it, the victim died from traumatic head injury. The dynamics of his fatal head injury explain his final hours. The haemorrhaging caused pressure on the brain with resultant swelling. The brain stem, located at the base of the brain, passes through a hole in the bottom of the skull, the *foramen magnum*. When the brain swells, the brain stem becomes pinched into this narrow passage way, causing it to stop functioning. When the brain stops functioning, the heart stops and death occurs.

From the initial blow, the clock began ticking until the brain stem swelled enough to shut down. What was the cause of death in this case? Was a fall or being hit cause a traumatic head injury? He could have lost consciousness or experienced a seizure brought on by his diabetic condition, or he could have passed out from excessive drinking, fallen and struck his head on something like the edge of a chair or coffee table.

Although no evidence of foul play was found, no skull fractures, no bruising on the scalp, no evidence of bruising on the inside of the scalp, enough doubt existed to rule the cause of death in this case as <u>undetermined</u>. The police were informed of the findings of the post-mortem, and they questioned the deceased's relatives and friends, although with little forensic evidence available, it would be difficult to prove homicide. However, the toxicology report revealed a key piece of evidence. A high blood-alcohol level indicated that the deceased could have drunk enough to pass out and his subsequent head injury resulting in an accidental death.

Road Traffic Death

The victim was a boy of nineteen who attempted to cross a busy road when he was struck by a car. Apparently he did not attempt to cross via the recognised pedestrian crossing, but instead darted in the middle of the road.

By his body, police found a pair of battered headphones and a CD player that he must have been wearing when the accident occurred. He did not see the car coming and the headphones would suggest he didn't hear it either. He was approximately six feet and one inches in height and weighed 171 pounds (approximately twelve stone).

Fatal vehicle accidents conjure up the image of a body battered, hammered into a pulp, but this is not always the case. The exterior of the victim's body showed evidence of just one injury, although more insidious ones must exist below the surface, because the superficial wound did not kill him. His lower leg contained a massive hole, the size of a cricket ball where something struck him with enormous force to split the skin and snap the tibia (shin bone). Strands of bright red muscle tissue protruded from the hole. Inside of it, one could see the fractured bone, bright white.

The open fracture on the victim's lower right leg was the probable point of impact. This wound probably occurred when the car's bumper struck the victim. An injury on the lower leg just above the ankle suggests that the car was braking when it struck him. When braking, momentum would cause the front of the vehicle to dip.

The various abrasions that covered the victim's body were catalogued for the post-mortem report. When investigating an accidental death, the pathologist needs to answer a number of questions. What killed the victim? Unless something unexpected surfaced – for example, the presence of a toxic substance in the victim's blood – the answer lay in the police accident report. What injuries did the victim suffer?

It is the post-mortem examination that will define the victim's injuries – evidence that can play a role in a potential civil action or criminal prosecution that may result from this tragic accident. A toxicology report revealing a substantial amount of a substance could potentially mitigate the driver's responsibility.

There was a bruise on the victim's lower right back, a wound resulting from a point of impact. When a large, heavy object such as a car travelling at 30-40 mph strikes a body, the fat underlying the point of impact often liquefies from the crushing effect of the car. On slicing into the bruise with a scalpel, under the skin is found partially liquefied fat, evidence of a glancing blow, but not the evidence for massive blunt force.

The car first struck the victim on another part of his body, most likely on his right shin. When the victim was rolled onto his side, his torso and legs moved, but his right lower leg did not, leaving the image of a lower leg twisted at a right-angle, exposing the bright white shin bone that partially protruded through the gaping hole left by the car's bumper. The victim's lungs contained bruising in the form of dark purple patches on the outer surface skin of the lungs. Two mechanisms could have caused this bruising; blunt force trauma to the chest or aspiration of blood.

A gouge in the lungs indicated that the victim also sustained rib fractures. The presence of the puncture suggests that some terrific force to his chest caused a fractured rib to jab into one of his lungs. The lung bruises could also have resulted from a second factor that might appear surprising.

114

Skull fractures cause bleeding inside the skull, during which sinuses drain blood into the throat. The victim will either spit out the blood or inhale it, and this blood often flows into the lungs, causing the bruised discoloured patches.

The victim's skull appeared like a cracked nutshell, several large fractures having created a criss-cross pattern. The fragmented skull suggests he took a massive hit. On examination, the brain is not the usual off-white colour, but crimson, mottled with haemorrhaging from being flooded with blood.

There were also tiny dots, red pin pricks which represented haemorrhaging around the blood vessels in the victim's brain. The brainstem contains nerve centres that control body functions. In this case, the brain sustained damage to these nerve centres, the accident destroying the control centre of the victim's brain. He would have died instantly. The extent of the damage to the skull indicated that he died on impact and most probably never knew what hit him. His head must have struck something with an edge, possible the force of the impact threw him onto the car's bonnet where he head struck the top edge of the windscreen. This victim died as a result of <u>massive head trauma</u>.

Gunshot Injury

The husband was startled by the sound of gunshot in an adjacent bedroom in his house. He told the police that he had found his wife inside the bedroom lying on her left side on a blood-spattered bed sheet, and a nine mm pistol lying on the bed in front of her. He picked up the gun, returned it to the bed and called the emergency services. He told detectives that his wife had been depressed since an accident a few years previously.

The victim appeared to have a single entrance

wound to the right temple between the eye and ear. However, two apparent exit wounds were visible on the left side of her head. This is a scenario that, while rare, does occur sometimes with 'jacked bullets' – these consist of a lead core with an outer copper jacket. When passing through the body, the core and jacket may separate causing individual exit wounds.

The pattern of gunpowder residue around a bullet entrance hole can tell the forensic pathologist the distance from which the fatal bullet was fired. A shotgun fired at a person's face from a few inches away would completely destroy the victim's face. A .22 pistol would leave a small neat bullet hole. If a precise estimate of range of fire is required, firearms examiners must test fire the weapon with the same type of ammunition used in the actual shooting. A tight contact wound (one that results when the gun is pressed against the head) with a smaller calibre weapon (9.22 or .25 calibre) may not cause splitting of the skin around the wound. The pattern of gunshot residue around the wound can indicate the distance between the pistol muzzle and in this case, the victim's head.

If, for instance, the pistol is pressed against the skull, the gases that discharge with the bullet have nowhere to escape but between the scalp and the skull, bursting the skin and creating a star-shaped wound around the entrance hole. This type of wound only occurs when the gun barrel is pressed against the skin that is stretched over bone, such as the skull and the sternum (breastbone).

Shots fired from less than an inch from the skull will leave a hole rimmed by residue including soot and partly burned flakes of gunpowder. A few inches more up to six inches away, the residue becomes like soot peppered around the entrance wound that may or may not, be driven into the skin, causing what is termed 'tattooing'. Because the many tiny black dots cannot be removed, the blast tattoos them onto the victim's scalp.

116

Suicide victims typically press the pistol tightly against the head or just a slight distance from the head, therefore the bullet wounds are characterised by singed, burned skin.

The entrance wound in this victim's head was a tight contact wound indicating that she pressed the gun against her head which is consistent with suicide victims, even though firearm suicides are less common among women than are suicides by other means.

On examination of the victim's body, no blood was found on her hands or arm even though the pistol had blood on it – strange for a victim who shot herself in the head.

While incising the victim's scalp in preparation for removing her brain, a second entrance wound in the right temple above her ear and behind the hairline was discovered. She had not been shot once, but twice in her right temple. The victim could not have shot herself in the head twice. The first wound would have left her comatose therefore an impossible suicide.

The post-mortem examination had turned up a concealed homicide. The first shot would have left the victim incapacitated instantaneously and given the placement of the first shot, she could not have then shot herself a second time. The existence of the second entrance wound proved that someone else must have been involved. With the cause of death listed as a homicide and supported by other independent forensic experts, the police launched a murder investigation.

Suspicion fell on her husband who discovered the body. Scenes of crime officers found tiny spots of blood on his shirt, and DNA testing confirmed the blood was that of the victim. A blood spatter expert examined the shirt the husband wore and the bed-sheets on which the victim was lying when she received the fatal wounds. The blood spatter that misted the bed-sheets exhibited a telltale pattern with a blank spot or shadow created by an obstruction, such as someone's outstretched arm.

A re-creation of the event confirmed this, and it was determined that the blood spatter patterns on the bed-sheets and on the husband's shirt, were consistent with someone standing over the victim and firing two shots into her head from a distance of just a few inches.

The tiny spots of blood found on the husband's shirt (under powerful lights using a magnifying glass) were caused by the mist of blood that, like a cloud, hovers around a victim immediately after the high-velocity impact of a bullet. These spots would appear on the shirt only if the person wearing it stood within four feet of the victim when the trigger was pulled.

This discovery by the forensic pathologist placed the husband inside the bedroom when the fatal shots were fired, not in an adjacent room as he had initially told police. Twelve months after the shooting, the husband stood trial for murder, was convicted and sentence to life-imprisonment.

Head Injury – Alcohol/Drug Overdose

The victim was a 26-year-old male who had hit his head a few times on the edge of a coffee table. After several cans of beer, he didn't feel any pain, and continued to play around with his friends until he collapsed and lost consciousness. He was rushed to the local hospital where he was pronounced dead on arrival. However, his distressed friends wondered, how did their party turn fatal?

The doctor who examined the victim on arrival at the hospital A&E department, performed a cursory external examination and performed a toxicology test. In the event that these tests fail to yield a sufficient cause of death, the victim will then be subject to a post-mortem examination.

The tests on this victim's blood revealed that he had consumed a substantial amount of alcohol the night he died.

He had a 24% (high) blood-alcohol level, and although this amount would not have killed him, it could, however, explain why he may have fallen and struck his head.

A preliminary examination, however, did not establish a cause of death. The key to this victim's death was probably the head injury. He hit his head harder than those at the party realised, and he sustained a fatal head injury. If he died of a head injury, it would be treated as accidental. If he died of something else, such as asphyxia, charges of manslaughter could be considered.

Having been found face-down, the post-mortem lividity had stained his head and face to a deep purple colouration.

An examination of his mouth revealed not teeth but nubs, the decayed remains of once healthy teeth. For the forensic pathologist, these rotten teeth represented evidence of a possible drug habit – likely *crystal methamphetamine.* Users and abusers often exhibit signs of poor hygiene such as rotten teeth, a condition sometimes referred to as 'meth-mouth'.

The post-mortem included another toxicology screening. The presence of 'meth' in the victim's blood could explain what occurred on the night in question. Use of this drug can lead to a stroke or cause the heart to beat erratically, which can lead to a fatal cardiac arrhythmia. Users of methamphetamine will often have scabs or sores on their bodies because the drug produces the feeling of bugs crawling on the skin.

A small hole, the circumference of a ballpoint pen, was found on the left side of the victim's chest. The hole represented a test done post-mortem during the initial examination at the hospital when the victim was first admitted. There was also a scrape on the left shoulder. A large number of pale red dots, broken blood vessels or petechiae are found on his back. These broken blood vessels are unlikely to have resulted from a crushing force applied to his torso. In this case, the broken blood vessels resulted from the lividity or settling of the blood after death.

Various fluids were collected from the body for toxicology testing; bile from the gallbladder to confirm, if necessary, blood levels of a drug; and fluid from the eye (vitreous humor) which was used to test for alcohol and other conditions such as diabetes.

There was no evidence of heart disease and thus, no reason to believe that the victim could have died from a heart attack.

There was no evidence of haemorrhage under the 'dura' membrane. Although the brain was swollen, he did not suffer from traumatic head injury or brain aneurysm that could have contributed to his death.

However, there was absence of sub-dural haematoma or bleeding under the 'dura' that would indicate he sustained a potentially lethal blow to the head. The internal examination revealed no other possible cause of death.

Test on the liver indicated that the victim suffered from neither alcoholism nor hepatitis-induced cirrhosis. Examination of stomach contents can provide a rough guide to the time of death. Generally, it takes about two hours for a meal to pass from the stomach to the small intestine. However, certain circumstances can impede digestion, such as stress. Examination of the brain revealed haemorrhages indicating that the victim hit his head but not hard enough to cause a lethal injury.

The results of the toxicology report proved that the victim's ultimate death resulted from a mixed drug intoxication; a combination of *oxycontin and alcohol.*

The Clapham Junction Railway Accident

On the rail lines running between Waterloo and Wimbledon in London, four rail tracks run through a 'cuttting' or embankment, about one mile west of Clapham Junction railway station. Peak hour trains passed through this cutting on a normal working morning at intervals of about two minutes.

Just after 8:00 am on Monday12 December, 1988, three trains were running towards this cutting. Two passengers trains on the Up Main Line were heading into Waterloo Station in the City, the third train had left Waterloo and was heading in the opposite direction towards Wimbledon on the adjoining Down Main Line.

The first passenger train travelling to Waterloo was the 7:18 from Basingstoke carrying twelve carriages. The second train was the 6:14 from Poole in Dorset, also carrying twelve carriages. The third train from Waterloo to Wimbledon was the 8:03 running empty of passengers.

At about 8:10 the driver of the Poole train, having passed signals at Green, was approaching the cutting. Having just taken a left-hand bend in the track, he saw immediately ahead of him, the Basingstoke train stationary on the same line with the signal at red. The distance was such that the Poole train could not possibly be stopped.

Despite emergency braking being applied, the front of the Poole train collided head-on into the rear of the stopped Basingstoke train. It was estimated that the Poole train would have been travelling at about 35 mph at the time of the impact.

The collision forced the Poole train to its off-side where it struck a glancing blow to the third empty train travelling towards Wimbledon and Haslemere. This blow derailed part of the third carriage of that train, but also kept the Poole train from moving further on its off-side and

121

finishing across the other tracks.

Local emergency services arrived at the scene in the cutting by 8:20 am. This was the beginning of an intensive rescue operation. The priority was to locate and evacuate the injured and the dead, together with the remainder of shocked crews and passengers who had managed to escape unscathed.

The 35 people, train crew and passengers who died as a result of the accident, had all been carried in the first two coaches of the Poole train, which were ripped open on their left-hand side. The leading coach of the Poole train suffered total disintegration on impact. The second coach, a trailer buffet car, had tables and chairs at its rear end. The buffet was not open on that particular day. The most seriously injured of the casualties were to be found in the first three carriages of the Poole train.

The rear coach of the first Basingstoke train was literally lifted in the air by the impact of the Poole train and ended up lying on its left side on the bank above the cutting wall. Its rear 'bogie' pierced the roof of the third coach of the Poole train. The next to the rear carriage of the Basingstoke train was derailed and came to rest, leaning against the embankment.

The rescue work was long and difficult, involving delicate lifting and cutting of wreckage in order to extricate those who were still trapped. It was only at 13:04 pm that the last casualty was evacuated to hospital and 15:45 pm before the last body was removed from the accident scene.

Thirty-three people died as a result of the accident, and two died later as a result of their injuries. Of the sixty-nine people who were seriously injured, many suffered permanent disablement. There were also 415 people who received minor injuries in the accident. The most obvious questions to be asked in an investigation of this magnitude are:

1. How had the accident happened?
2. How had the signalling system failed?

The answer to the first question was that is it was caused by a signalling failure, and to the second, during alterations to the signalling system, a wire should have been removed, in error it was not. It was still in the system and was making an electrical contact with its old circuit. It was, therefore, able to feed current into the new system when that current should have been dead. It was this current that prevented the signal in question from turning to red.

The Post-Mortem Pathology Report from Dr Iain West, Forensic Pathologist

It was several hours before all the bodies of those killed in the crash were delivered to Westminster Mortuary. In charge of the pathology team was Dr Iain West, assisted by Dr Richard Shepherd.

Each of the bodies was identified by means of personal possessions; clothing, jewellery, documents etc. Fingerprints and blood/tissue samples were taken and dental charting made. Each body was then given an identification number. To compound the difficult situation, the forensic pathologists did not have the opportunity to attend the actual scene of the disaster before the bodies of those killed had been removed from the scene. This prevented photographs being taken of the bodies *in situ*.

By noting the positions of the bodies, this would have assisted in the task of reconstructing the accident. In rail disasters, there are serious problems in identifying victims, and in accessing exactly how many passengers were travelling in the trains at the time. This difficulty was compounded at Clapham when it was realised that there were about 62 body parts retrieved from the mangled wreckage. The post-mortem reports into the fatalities record a variety of horrendous injuries, the majority being classed as 'severe blunt force injuries'.

In the case of one male passenger, the report recorded:

> "Traumatic amputation of the head and upper neck. Amputation of the right upper limb at shoulder level. Amputation of the left thigh about the pelvis, with amputation of the right leg at knee level. There were multiple lacerations on the scalp; multiple areas of bruising and abrasions on the face, the trachea and neck. Vessels protruding from the amputated ends appeared to be cleanly incised. There were extensive crush-type abrasions over the whole of the upper chest. The deceased had suffered severe mutilation injuries, as a result of being trapped within the deforming wreckage of the front of the first carriage. He could well have been standing and then subsequently suffered the extensive dismemberment after being struck by parts of the super-structure of the carriage. His other injuries were caused by his body being pulled under the wreckage by the force of the impact".

Another case was reported:

> "The pattern of injury shows severe crush injuries to the trunk, a violent impact to the head, and injury to the lower limbs. This appears to be typical of the patterns seen in passengers who had been ejected from their seats following the collision, with the head impacting against a hard surface. Leg injuries

appear to result from entrapment of the legs as
the floor and seats deformed. The crush injuries
to the chest are likely to be the result of
propulsion of the body, combined with the
subsequent crushing by debris".

A further case of a man who died of traumatic asphyxia
was reported:
"The appearance indicated he had suffered
severe compression of the chest and upper
abdomen, as a consequence of being crushed by
debris. The absence of severe trauma suggests
that he was compressed by relatively soft-
surfaced objects, suggesting that he was seated
at the time of the impact".

According to Dr West, the main pathological findings were:
"Out of seventy-one passengers travelling in the
first carriage of the 'Poole' train, twenty-nine died. It
transpires that the front nearside of this carriage was the
most dangerous, no one escaped either death or severe
injury in this area. There were forty-three passengers in the
second carriage of the 'Poole' train which served as a buffet
car. All the passengers who died in this carriage were
seated, two were on the offside and four on the nearside of
the carriage which suffered severe damage. All but one of
the victims are thought to have been seated at the time of
the collision. The medical evidence as deduced from the
pattern of injuries, would support this view. Seventeen
passengers were in seats in the front compartment of the
first carriage. From the patterns of injuries suffered by
many, it is possible that most of the twelve passengers were
seated either at the very front of the carriage, or in nearside
rows of seats. Injuries to victims who were placed in the
front carriage showed two main patterns. Those at the front
suffered severe crushing injuries caused by destruction of

the front of the train on impact. Further injuries were caused by ejection from the seats at the time of the impact. Much of the mutilating injury suffered by the victims in this part of the train was due to post-mortem damage caused by their bodies being drawn into the wreckage as the buffet car rolled over the front carriage.

The heavy toll among passengers seated at the rear nearside of the train, appears to have resulted from forceful impact in that part of the carriage. They suffered severe primary impact, mainly to the side of the head and or trunk, which was adjacent to the window. Lower limb injuries, frequently of great severity, were also common among the passengers seated on the nearside of the carriage due to their legs being trapped and crushed by the wreckage of the seats. Traumatic or crush asphyxia was not a common cause of death among passengers killed in the first carriage. However, one passenger suffered asphyxial damage caused by ejection from her seat and being thrown so that her neck struck a hard surface. All six victims killed in the buffet car, appeared to have been seated at the tables. Three of these died from traumatic asphyxia caused by tables being forced back into the chest and abdomen. Marks on the bodies were consistent with pressure from the tables".

Sources: Dr Iain West's Casebook, Chester Stern (Warner Books, London, 1997, pp 163-174). Investigation into the Clapham Junction Railway Accident, Anthony Hidden QC (Department of Transport, HMSO London, 1989).

Medical Detectives: Pioneering Forensic Pathologists

"The development of forensic medicine in Britain is told through the lives of the five great pathologists who dominated the scene throughout most of the twentieth century. Spanning seventy years, their careers and achievements marked major milestones in the development of legal medicine, their work and innovation laying the foundations for modern crime scene investigation (CSI). Sir Bernard Spilsbury, Sir Sydney Smith, and Professors John Glaister, Francis Camps and Keith Simpson, were the original expert witnesses. Between them, they performed over 200,000 post-mortems during their professional careers, establishing crucial elements of murder investigation, such as time, place and cause of death. This forensic quintet featured in many notable murder trials of their time, making ground-breaking discoveries in the process. The five pathologists, each with their unique talents, represented a golden age of forensic development. Their careers overlapped to a considerable extent and there were strains of rivalry in their relationships at times. This was perhaps, inevitable in the adversarial system employed in British courts, which meant that experts were sometimes cast as opponents in the courtroom. As professionals, they did not always agree in the interpretation of evidence. Despite their differences, they elevated the gritty, not to say, gruesome business of examining the dead, to a multi-faceted profession, calling on every available scientific resource and discipline. Crime scene investigation as it is practised today, owes a great deal to these pioneers for their questioning spirit and innovative genius".

Professor Bernard Knight, CBE

Sir Bernard Spilsbury (1877-1947)

Sir Bernard Spilsbury was an iconic figure who put forensic pathology on the map with his involvement in the Crippen Case in 1910. He was, in essence, a loner; an interpreter who exemplified the role of the expert witness. Sure of himself, certain of the facts and not requiring a second opinion, he stood tall in the witness box.

In an age when capitol punishment was still in use, his courtroom testimony made him an arbiter of life and death. A roll call of his cases reads like a catalogue of famous British murders. His conclusions though, were often controversial and contested and remain so to this day. He was the epitome of the expert, aloof, assured and respected.

Sir Sydney Smith (1883-1969)

Spilsbury's contemporary, Sir Sydney Smith by contrast, was an innovator, a clubbable man who worked on a broad canvas and drew people towards him. Born in New Zealand, he pursued his training in Scotland, the spiritual home of forensic medicine. He honed his skills in Egypt where he worked during the inter-war years, and pioneered the development of forensic ballistics. He returned to Edinburgh to concentrate on teaching and helped to put forensic studies onto a sound academic basis.

John Glaister (1892-1971)

John Glaister also prospered in the Scottish tradition and played a major role in furthering his nation's pre-eminent position in forensic medicine. He was a professor for thirty years at Glasgow University where he succeeded his father. His particular contribution was to apply scientific methods to the examination of trace evidence gleaned at crime scenes. His work on the identification of hair was a significant breakthrough, and like Smith, he was willing to share knowledge and to call for specialist help when it was needed. This was evident in the Ruxton case when he pioneered photo-imposition as an identification technique.

Francis Camps (1905-1972)

Francis Camps was an organiser rather than an innovator. He had a vision of co-ordinating the emerging skills of the broader medico-legal profession and, to that end, created a world-class forensic department at London University. He had his share of important crime cases, but was at his best when managing people and resources to advance the knowledge and professional status of forensic work. He was a founding member of the British Academy of Forensic Sciences, which succeeded in bringing science, medicine and the law together to serve the ends of justice. Camps also reached out to the USA to add an international element to what he viewed as best practice.

Keith Simpson (1907-1985)

Keith Simpson combined a number of talents as teacher and practitioner. He was also an important innovator breaking new ground in the understanding of factors which determined time of death, and helped to put forensic dentistry on the map as a means of establishing identity. Like his contemporaries, he was involved in many headline murder cases, Heath, Haigh and Christie being prominent among them. He was a highly effective communicator, noted for his succinct delivery of evidence in court, in addition to his lecturing and writing activities.
Source: The History Press - The Destination for History - Author: Robin Odell.

Glossary of Medical Terms

To the layperson, medical terminology can appear like a foreign language and difficult to understand. However, the key to understanding these terms is to focus on their component parts (prefixes, roots and suffixes). For example, *dermato* refers to the 'skin'. Therefore the medical specialism *dermatology* refers to the study and treatment of skin conditions.

Knowing the meaning of a small number of these components, can help with interpreting a much larger number of common medical terms. The following list defines the most commonly used medical terms.

Acou	Hear
Actyl	Finger/toe
Aden	Gland
Aer	Air
Alg	Pain
Andro	Man
Angio	Vessel
Ankyl	Crooked or curved
Ante	Before
Anter	Front or forward
Anti	Against
Arterio	Artery
Arthro	Joint
Articul	Joint
Athero	Fatty
Audio	Hearing
Auri	Ear
Bi	Double/two
Brachy	Short
Brady	Slow
Bucco	Cheek

Carcino	Cancer
Cardi	Heart
Cephal	Head
Cerebro	Brain
Cervic	Neck
Chandr(o)	Cartilage
Chol(e)	Bile/gall bladder
Circum	Around
Contra	Against
Corpor	Body
Costo	Rib
Crani	Skull
Cryo	Cold
Cut	Skin
Cyan	Blue
Cysto	Bladder
Cyto	Cell
Dent	Tooth
Diplo	Double
Dors	Black
Dys	Bad/abnormal
Ectomy	Excision by cutting
Emia	Blood
Encephalo	Brain
Endo	Inside
Epi	Outer
Erythro	Red
Extra	Outside
Gastro	Stomach
Gen	Originate (as in Genesis)
Glosso	Tongue
Glyco	Sweet/glucose
Gram	Write/record
Gyn	Woman
Hemato	Blood
Hemi	Half

Hepat	Live
Histo	Tissue
Ophthalmo	Eye
Hydro	Water
Hyper	High/excessive
Hypo	Low/deficient
Hystero	Uterus
Infra	Beneath
Inter	Between
Intra	Inside
Itis	Inflammation
Lacto	Milk
Laparo	Abdomen
Latero	Side
Leuko	White
Linguo	Tongue
Lipo	Fat
Pharmaco	Drug
Lysis	Dissolve
Pharyngo	Throat
Mal	Abnormal/bad
Malac	Soft
Mammo	Breast
Masto	Breast
Megalo	Large
Melano	Black
Meningo	Membranes
Pneumono	Lung
Myco	Fungus
Myo	Muscle
Naso	Nose
Necro	Death
Nephro	Kidney
Neuro	Nerve
Nutri	Nourish
Oculo	Eye

Odyno	Pain
Oma	Tumour
Onco	Tumour
Opia	Vision
Opsy	Examination (autopsy)
Orchio	Testes
Osis	Condition
Osseo	Bone
Osteo	Bone
Oto	Ear
Patho	Disease
Pedo	Child
Penia	Deficient
Pepto	Digest
Peri	Around
Phago	Destroy
Phlebo	Vein
Phobia	Fear
Plasty	Repair
Plegia	Paralysis
Pnea	Breathing
Pneumato	Breath/air
Podo	Foot
Poly	Many/much
Post	After
Poster	Behind / back
Procto	Anus
Psendo	False
Psycho	Mind
Pulmono	Lung
Pyelo	Pelvis of kidney
Pyro	Fever/fire
Rachi	Spine
Reno	Kidneys
Rhag	Break/burst
Rhe	Flow

Rhino	Nose
Sclero	Hard
Scope	Instrument
Scopy	Examination
Somato	Body
Spondy	Vertebra
Steat	Fat
Steno	Narrow/compressed
Stetho	Chest
Stom	Opening
Supra	Above
Tachy	Fast/quick
Therap	Treatment
Thermo	Heat
Thorac	Chest
Throm	Clot/lump
Tomy	Incision (operation by cutting)
Toxi	Poison
Uria	Urine
Vacso	Vessel
Veno	Vein
Vesico	Bladder

Selected Bibliography

ERZINCLIOGLU, Z *Maggots, Murder and Men*, (Harley Books, Colchester, 2000)

FERNER, RE *Forensic Pharmacology: Medicine, Mayhem and Malpractice,* (Oxford Medical Publications, Oxford, 1996)

FRAZER, J & WILKES, R (Eds) *The Handbook of Forensic Science Investigation* (Willan, 2009)

GARRETT, G & NOTT, A *Causes of Death,* (Constable & Robinson, London, 2001)

KNIGHT, B *Simpson's Forensic Medicine*, (Edward Arnold, London, 1991)

LICHTENBERG, W 'Methods for the Determination of Shooting Distance,'*Forensic Science Review,* 1990 2, 37-44

MASON, JK *The Pathology of Violent Injury,* (Edward Arnold, London, 1978)

Mc DERMID, V *Forensics: The Anatomy of Crime,* (Profile Books, London, 2015)

ROACH, M *Stuff: The Curious Lives of Human Cadavers*, (Viking, London, 2003)

ROSE, M *Lethal Witness: Sir Bernard Spilsbury, Honorary Pathologist*, (Stroud, Sutton, 2007)

ROBERTSON, B & VIGNAUX, GA *Interpreting Evidence: Evaluating Forensic Evidence in the Court Room*, (Wiley, Chichester, 1995)

SAUKKO, P & KNIGHT, B (Eds) *Knight's Forensic Pathology*, (Hodder Arnold, London, 2004)

SIMPSON, K *Forty Years of Murder*, (Granada Publishing, London, 1981)

SMITH, S *Mostly Murder,* (Harrap, London, 1986)

STERN, C *Dr Iain West's Casebook*, (Little Brown, London, 1996)

VANEZIS, P & BURSTILL, A *Suspicious Death Scene Investigation*, (Oxford University Press, 1996)

WARLOW, TA *Firearms, the Law and Forensic Ballistics* (Taylor & Francis, 2004)

WHITE, PC (Eds) *Crime Scene to Court: Essentials of Forensic Science,* (Society of Chemistry, Cambridge, 1998)

WILKINSON, F *Firearms*, (Camden House, London, 1977)

Printed in Great Britain
by Amazon

46813801R00076